CARDIOLOGY RESEARCH AND CLINICAL DEVELOPMENTS

CARDIAC REHABILITATION IN WOMEN

CARDIOLOGY RESEARCH
AND CLINICAL DEVELOPMENTS

Additional books in this series can be found on Nova's website at:

https://www.novapublishers.com/catalog/index.php?cPath=23_29&seriesp
=Cardiology%20Research%20and%20Clinical%20Developments
&sort=2a&page=1

Additional e-books in this series can be found on Nova's website at:

https://www.novapublishers.com/catalog/index.php?cPath=23_29&seriesp
e=Cardiology+Research+and+Clinical+Developments

CARDIOLOGY RESEARCH AND CLINICAL DEVELOPMENTS

CARDIAC REHABILITATION IN WOMEN

ARZU DAŞKAPAN

Nova Science Publishers, Inc.
New York

NOTICE TO THE READER

The Publisher has taken reasonable care in the preparation of this book, but makes no expressed or implied warranty of any kind and assumes no responsibility for any errors or omissions. No liability is assumed for incidental or consequential damages in connection with or arising out of information contained in this book. The Publisher shall not be liable for any special, consequential, or exemplary damages resulting, in whole or in part, from the readers' use of, or reliance upon, this material. Any parts of this book based on government reports are so indicated and copyright is claimed for those parts to the extent applicable to compilations of such works.

Independent verification should be sought for any data, advice or recommendations contained in this book. In addition, no responsibility is assumed by the publisher for any injury and/or damage to persons or property arising from any methods, products, instructions, ideas or otherwise contained in this publication.

This publication is designed to provide accurate and authoritative information with regard to the subject matter covered herein. It is sold with the clear understanding that the Publisher is not engaged in rendering legal or any other professional services. If legal or any other expert assistance is required, the services of a competent person should be sought. FROM A DECLARATION OF PARTICIPANTS JOINTLY ADOPTED BY A COMMITTEE OF THE AMERICAN BAR ASSOCIATION AND A COMMITTEE OF PUBLISHERS.

LIBRARY OF CONGRESS CATALOGING-IN-PUBLICATION DATA

Daskapan, Arzu.
  Cardiac rehabilitation in women / Arzu Daskapan.
    p. ; cm.
  Includes bibliographical references and index.
  ISBN 978-1-61668-146-3 (softcover)
  1. Heart diseases in women. 2. Heart--Diseases--Patients--Rehabilitation.
I. Title.
  [DNLM: 1. Cardiovascular Diseases--rehabilitation. 2. Cardiovascular
Diseases--epidemiology. 3. Risk Factors. 4. Sex Factors. 5. Women's
Health. WG 166 D229c 2010]
  RC682.D34 2010
  616.1'20082--dc22
                                                              2010002976

Published by Nova Science Publishers, Inc. ✤ New York

CONTENTS

PREFACE

Diagnostic and treatment methods in the field of health care continue to improve. As a result of these improvements, chronic disease-related deaths somewhat declined and life expectancy increased. However, the burden of cardiovascular disease world-wide has become one of great concern to patients and health care agencies alike. Circulatory diseases, including myocardial infarction and stroke, kill more people than any other disease.

Also, cardiovascular diseases remain the leading cause of deaths and disabilities in women. Cardiac rehabilitation programs are critically important in reducing recurrent cardiovascular events, to improve survival and enhance quality of life. It is known that women's participation and adherence rates to cardiac rehabilitation are low. On the other hand, there are gender differences in the recognition, diagnosis, treatment, and outcomes for patients with cardiovascular diseases and most of them are perhaps disadvantageous to women. When these reports were examined, the results had shown that the number of deaths related to cardiovascular diseases for females has exceeded those for males and it continues to rise.

Women are considered the foundation in family life. Today, the women have many family-related responsibilities, as well as actively work and contribute to society's productivity. If a woman has any chronic disease such as heart disease, all family members are negatively affected by her illness. Also, cardiovascular diseases in women impose a significant social and economic burden on health services in many countries. Protection for women against cardiovascular disease is very important for public health promotion. At the same time, there is need for increasing popularity of cardiac rehabilitation programs among female cardiac patients.

This book tries to summarize how "being female" may impact on cardiac rehabilitation. In this sense, the text helps to:

- increase recognition to address the need for heart health protection and promotion for women
- make women conscious of cardiovascular diseases and possible future complications
- to better understand gender differences related to cardiovascular diseases in women
- design more cardiac rehabilitation programs based on a woman's individual socioeconomic characteristics, clinical profile and concerns.

Hopefully, this soft cover book will aid to reach these goals and will help health care professionals develop the problem-solving skills to manage female patients with cardiovascular diseases.

Arzu Daşkapan
Ankara, 2009

Chapter 1

WOMEN AND PREVALENCE
OF CARDIOVASCULAR DISEASES

The term cardiovascular disease (CVD) includes diseases of the heart and blood vessel system and is usually related to atherosclerosis [1]. Over the last few decades, CVD has become the leading cause of death and disability worldwide [2, 3]. Breast cancer was thought as the greatest health concern for women [4]. Research has indicated that myocardial infarction (MI), stroke and related CVD are responsible for almost twice as many deaths among women than all forms of cancer combined [5]. Unfortunately, CVD has higher death rates, more recurrent episodes, and more frequent cause of hospital admission in women than in men [6]. In Europe, more women than men die in consequence of heart disease [7]. In the United States, 54% of total CVD deaths are women by comparison to only 46% for men [8]. Data in England has shown that coronary heart disease is responsible from almost 114,000 deaths a year and one in six are women [9]. Previous studies revealed the proportion of CVD deaths in Turkey increased from 20% in 1960 to 40-50 % in 1990 [10]; and contrary to expectations the coronary morbidity and mortality in premenopausal Turkish women approaches that of Turkish men [11]. New Zealand Ministry of Health reported that CVD accounted for 25.4 % of male, and 21.1 % of female deaths and the burden of disease resulting from CVD is high [12]. In Australia, CVD is a major cause of morbidity in women [13]. Recently, one review study introduced CVD as the primary cause of deaths in Indian, Chinese, and Saudi women [14]. It seems evident that heart disease is a serious health problem for women in different countries around the world. On the other hand, the burden of CVD on global economy is great. Therefore, health policies for the prevention of heart disease have not lost popularity in the different countries around the world.

Chapter 2

RISK FACTORS FOR CARDIOVASCULAR DISEASE IN WOMEN

A report published in 2001 in the Institute of Medicine clearly indicated there is a need for the evaluation of sex-based differences in human disease and medical research, and to incorporate these differences into clinical practice [16]. There are major differences between women and men regarding pathophysiology, clinical presentation, diagnostic strategies, response to therapies, and adverse outcomes of CVD [17].

It is well demonstrated that certain risk factors play a role in the development and progression of CVD. Inter Heart Study determined nine factors that are responsible for 90% all cases of CVD. These are dyslipidaemia, hypertension, smoking stress, diabetes, obesity (especially abdominal fat distrubition), physical inactivity, poor diet and excessive alcohol consumption [18]. Traditional cardiac risk factors are essentially the same for men and women, but there are important quantitative differences between these two genders. Women have smaller artery dimension, different electrical properties, and different plaque composition and development [19]. One research reported that the left main coronary artery and the left anterior descending artery are smaller in women, and the smaller lumen may be the cause of arterial occlusion in the presence of relatively small plaque [20].

The major identified risk factors for CVD in women are tobacco use, hypertension, diabetes mellitus, dyslipidemia, obesity, sedentary lifestyle, and atherogenic diet [21]. More recently identified risk factors in women include high sensitivity C-reactive protein (CRP), homocysteine, and lipoprotein (a) [22].

The CRP protein is found in the blood, the protein levels rise in response to inflammation [23]. The role of elevated basal levels of CRP in cardiovascular disease was demonstrated among healthy men; later it was shown that CRP predicts vascular events even among low-risk subgroups of women with no readily apparent markers for disease. [24, 25]

One comprehensive review revealed elevated lipoprotein (a) levels are strongly related to CVD events than to severity of coronary artery disease in both women and men [26].

Men have generally less favorable cardiac risk factors than women; on the other hand, it was found that some risk factors (diabetes mellitus, hypertension, smoking, hypercholesterolemia, and obesity) were more important for CVD in female coronary patients [27,28].

Diabetes increases CVD risk as a 3-7-fold in women compared to a 2-3-fold elevation of risk in men. Diabetes negates the presumed gender-protective effect of estrogen in premenopausal women [29]. According to estimates two-thirds of all diabetic deaths are due to CVD [6].

Hypertension is more prevalent in women than in men after the age of 65. It was proven that three out of four women with hypertension are aware of the problem but only one in three will take any action to control it [30]. Contrary to earlier belief, women do not tolerate the effects of hypertension on cardiovascular and renal system better than men [31]. Blood pressure of <120/80mmHg should be maintained by women. It was observed that there was a threefold increase in CVD among women with systolic blood pressure >185 mmHg as compared with women with blood pressure <135 mmHg [32].

It was indicated that smoking is the leading cause of CVD in women younger than 50 years. The prevalence of smokers is still slightly higher in men than in women, but the decline in tobacco use among women is less evident than in men [33]. Based on some previous reports; smoking is a risk factor for women even if they smoke only two to five cigarettes daily [34-36]. One previous study has shown that even light smokers (1- 4 cigarettes/day) had twice the risk of a nonfatal myocardial infarction or CHD death than nonsmokers [37]. Negative effects of smoking on lipid profile are more prominent in women than in men [38]. The risk in young female smokers is additionally elevated by the use of oral contraceptives [39].

Dyslipidemia profile in women is different from men in CVD development [26]. There is a linear relationship between low-density lipoprotein levels and risk for CVD particularly in women less than 65 years. Additionally, low high-density lipoprotein levels in women over 65 years convey a greater risk than in men [6, 40]. HDL-C is entitled as "good cholesterol" [41].

Large cohort studies have demonstrated that high density lipoprotein cholesterol levels are a strong, independent inverse predictor of CVD [42, 43]. Low HDL-C value was defined as less than 40 mg/dL [44]. Obesity, cigarette smoking, and a sedentary lifestyle may cause low blood levels of HDL [45]. Lifestyle modification may help to raise HDL-C [41]. Former studies found that each increase of 1 mg per deciliter (0.03 mmol per liter) in HDL cholesterol is associated with a decrease of 2 to 3% in the risk of future coronary heart disease [46]. Skoumas *et al.* study demonstrated that for women the dose response relationship between physical activity and HDL cholesterol levels can be a positive indicator. [47].

Obesity is a common risk factor for CVD in men and women; however, several prospective studies have shown that obesity may be a greater risk factor for women [48]. Obesity increases the CVD risk in women and is associated with diabetes, hypertension, and dyslipidemia; as well as other lifestyle-related risk factors such as physical inactivity and bad diet [27, 49]. Central obesity is associated with insulin resistance, so it is even more hazardous [50].

Oral contraceptive use, menopause, and hormone replacement therapy use are gender-specific cardiovascular risk factors in women [51].

One review study reported that older oral contraceptives contained high doses of estrogen and increased risk for cardiovascular disease but modern oral contraceptives have one fourth of the estrogen and one tenth of the progestogen. Also this review stated that compared to older oral contraceptives, newer ones have lower risk for cardiovascular disease [52].

More recent study demonstrated that hormone therapy increases risk for a recurrent coronary event in the short term and that hormone therapy should not be initiated solely for prevention of recurrent heart disease [53].

Distribution of CVD risk factors in women may vary from country to country. It was indicated: 23.4% of women were diabetic, 60.3% were hypertensive, and 59.7% had histories of hyperlipidemia, and 9.2% smoked in United States [54]. Based on the literature, compared to white women; CVD risk levels were more remarkable among black women with higher prevalence of hypertension, obesity, diabetes, and stress [55]. Also reported, Turkish women have higher blood cholesterol levels; hypertension, diabetes and body mass index than men [56]. One study completed in Iran, showed the prevalence of hypertension and diabetes mellitus significantly higher in Iranian women [57]. Sasaki *et al.* reported that the incidence of coronary events was 60% lower in Japanese women than in men. Although the correlation of serum total cholesterol and low-density lipoprotein cholesterol concentrations to coronary events were similar in Japanese men and women, the low-density lipoprotein cholesterol concentration associated with a decreased risk of coronary events was slightly higher in women. Diabetes mellitus was a stronger risk factor in Japanese women than in men [58]. In China, the age-standardized prevalence rates of dyslipidemia and hypertension in women 35 to 74 years of age are 53% and 25%, respectively [59].

Since the late 1950s, the role of potential psychosocial risk factors had been mentioned in the development of CVD. These are Type A personality (excesses of aggression, hurry, and competitiveness) and more recently type D personality (inhibition of negative emotions in social situations), depression and anxiety, low socioeconomic status, lack of social support, social isolation and chronic work stress [27]. It has been proven that low socioeconomic status as defined by occupational position, income, or education is a major psychosocial risk factor in both men and women. It was demonstrated that there are gender differences in the importance of these factors [60,61]. For example, based on some reports, type A behavior was more related to the increased CVD risk in males than in females [62, 63]. On the other hand, less than 8 years of education contributed to a 4-fold risk of women (compared with women with 12 and more years of education) of developing CVD over a 14-year [64].

This indicated that for both work-related and home-related life events the affected risk increase in females [60, 61, 65]. Family-related stress is important factor for women's cardiovascular health [66]. It was found that marital stress enhanced the risk of recurrent coronary events and death among women [67]. Blom *et al.* research found that marital stress also had negatively affected social relations among middle-aged women with CVD [68]. Unlike women, men are influenced by only work-related occasions [60, 61, 65].

Hallman *et al.* confirmed that women appear to be more sensitive than men with respect to psychosocial risk factors for CVD. According to their findings; the relative sensitivity of work content, workload and control, physical stress reactions, emotional stress reactions, and burnout were higher for women than for men [69].

Beckie *et al.* examined physiological and psychosocial profiles of 182 women. This study found that although physiological profiles were similar, younger women had significantly worse psychosocial profiles than older women; and depressive symptoms and anxiety were more prevalent, more serious in younger women. CR team should provide efficacious interventions to improve the psychosocial health for women with heart disease. [70].

Various studies about coronary risk factors have been carried out to ensure successful life style modifications. One study assessed the relationships between the patients' beliefs about the causes of their heart disease, risk factors, sex and socioeconomic status. This study's findings were interesting. Men were more likely than women to attribute heart disease to smoking, poor diet, and working too hard, but more women than men believed that chance or bad luck was responsible [71].

When the results of these studies concerning coronary risk factors in women were interpreted as holistically; it is obvious that their needs require different solutions than men to address the risk factor management among healthy women or women with heart disease.

Chapter 3

MENOPAUSE AND CVD

The transition to menopause is a complex physiological process of women's life, often accompanied by the additional effects of aging and social adjustment [72]. Also, menopause should be considered as an important period for heart disease prevention in women. Mostly, CVD is not observed in premenopausal females, especially non-smokers [73]. Incidence of cardiovascular events increases most markedly after the age of 45–54 years (i.e., at the time of the menopause) [74]. Incidence of MI is high in women who undergo menopause [75]. These increases in cardiac events suggest that endogenous reproductive hormones have likely a protective effect.

Effects of menopause may vary depending on menopausal age. More serious health problems may develop in women who experience early menopause. Early menopause increases lifetime risk of death from ischemic heart disease [76].

It was suggested that some factors have been contributed to an early onset of natural menopause. A consistent finding is that smoking is associated with occurrence of spontaneous early menopause [77, 78]. Some studies have reported a dose-response effect of smoking on early menopause [79,80]. On the other hand, it was shown that there was relationship between active smoking and early menopause [80-82].

Other factors include race [83], low income [84], body-mass index [83], nulliparity [85], being single [84, 86], depression [87], and genetic factors [78-86]

Menopause results from reduced secretion of the ovarian hormones estrogen and progesterone [72]. Around menopause, estrogen levels decline by 80% [39]. It is known that ovarian hormones protects against CVD. In menopausal stage, loss of ovarian function is associated with adverse metabolic changes [73, 88].

Total cholesterol and low-density lipoprotein cholesterol increased; high-density lipoprotein slightly decreased [89]. This determined that dyslipidemiais is associated with increased oxidative stress and endothelial dysfunction [90]. Following menopause insulin sensitivity decreased with time and insulin response to a glucose challenge [91]. There is central body fat accumulation and change in body composition [92, 93]. There is a reduction in fibrinolytic activity following the menopause, and no reduction or slight increase in coagulant activity and as a result tipped towards coagulation [94]. After menopause, the increase in arterial pressure in women is such that the prevalence of hypertension is higher in postmenopausal women than in age-matched men [95]. All of these changes may explain why postmenopausal women have higher CVD risk than premenopausal women.

At the same time, menopause leads to sedentary life style by diminishing effort tolerance and peak oxygen consumption in women [96]. It was thought that endothelium-dependent dysfunction may be responsible for these changes [97] because ovarian hormone deficiency affects negatively vessel-wall physiology [98]. As a result of these impairments, even healthy postmenopausal women may complain of fatigue at rest and during exercise [99, 100]. To emphasize that during the menopausal period an active life style that includes regular exercise is essential for CVD risk factor management. Despite lower exercise tolerance issues, it is important to build exercise habit to post- menopausal women. However, some precautions should be taken for safe exercise such as monitorization, and supervision by experienced health care professional.

On the other hand, rates of depression are high among postmenopausal women. It is evident that depression causes a greater increase in CVD incidence in women and often female CVD patients experience higher levels of depression than men [27].

A history of depressive disorders, poor physical heath and life stressors (lack of employment and social support), history of surgical menopause, and a long perimenopausal transition are some of risk factors for the development of depression during the perimenopausal period. [101]. Regular exercise may also help to improve the depression.

Chapter 4

GENDER DIFFERENCES RELATED TO CVD IN WOMEN

There are biological and gender inequalities in diagnosis, treatment, prevention, and rehabilitation of ischemic heart disease [102]. The developments have been obtained in drug therapy and control of cardiovascular risk factors in women in recent years, but compared to men; improvements in survival in women did not reach desired levels [103].

Because of biological differences between the sexes; it was established that were some disparities in the utilization of health care services. One old study's found that women are more likely to need medical care for anemia, diabetes, osteoarthritis and rheumatoid arthritis, but men seem to have higher rates of heart disease, hypertension and cholesterol problems [104]. It seems, from the 1980's until today, women did not raise awareness about the seriousness of heart disease.

The prognosis is worse for women than men [105]. After MI, women's short-term and long-term outcomes were worst than the men's [106, 107]. The rate of return to work after MI or CABG is significantly lower in women than in men [108]. One study reported that the 1-year mortality after MI is higher in women than in men [109].

Compared to men, CVD in women is developed later in life [110]. Among women, onset age is 10 years older and first MI time is probably 20 years older than men. This probability or thought related to late onset brings about difficulties in the prevention of CVD among young or middle-aged women: these women do not attach importance to this subject and postpone taking measurements against the disease [111,112]. At the same time, advanced age is associated with higher possibility of morbid factors such as diabetes mellitus, hypertension, hypercholesterolemia, peripheral vascular disease, and heart failure. These factors may play a role in the worse prognosis among women with heart disease [112-114]. Later onset of CVD seems likely to be more disadvantageous rather than advantageous for women.

Symptoms of CVD tend to display itself differently in women than in men. Atypical and non-chest pain presentations are more common in women, to the extent that it has been suggested that clinical presentation and risk factor analysis are of less value in predicting CVD for women than for men [115]. For example, chest pain is the most common presenting symptom of acute MI, however women may have atypical symptoms such as back pain, burning in the chest, abdominal discomfort, nausea, shortness of breath or fatigue.

In the late myocardial infarction period, Q-waves are observed on the electrocardiogram in men. But women may not have Q-waves present and they are more likely to demonstrate nondiagnostic, reversible ST segment elevations or T-wave abnormalities [116].

Misdiagnosis is common in women [112, 117, 118]. Existence of some previous disease, such as arthritis, peptic ulcer disease, or chronic lung disease may cause more confusion regarding symptoms and a missed diagnosis in the event of an acute MI [119]. The quality of the chest pain or discomfort in women is usually less severe and or milder compared to men [118]. So 50% of MI's are unrecognized in women versus 33% in men [120]. More striking is the result that two thirds of women who die suddenly from heart disease had no previously recognized symptoms [121]. Early symptom recognition, prompt diagnosis and immediate treatment should be given to importance in women [1].

Many women thought their symptoms as insignificant [4]. Research reported that, women may value the health and/or well-being of others in their families over themselves [122-124]. Women are aware of delaying symptom assessment and disease treatment to accommodate family needs [123]. Mostly women are not disposed to seek medical help or to further examine their disease, and often under these conditions postpone hospital attention t for effective treatment [112]. It has been considered that this lack of aggressive management toward these early symptoms may be responsible for the higher mortality rate in women [51]. Studies' findings show that women arrive an hour later to the hospital on the average, progress to more severe conditions and have a greater risk of adjusted mortality at 28 days [125]. Especially young women (< 55 years) have a worse prognosis from acute MI than their male counterparts, with a greater recurrence of MI and higher mortality [106-126].

A recent review concluded that there is limited data on whether many established tests and procedures are appropriate for women [127].

The differences in clinical presentation and the lower prevalence of obstructive CVD complicate the diagnosis of CVD in women [128, 129]. There is need for an effective diagnostic strategy for women at risk because up to 40% of initial cardiac events are fatal [130]. A consensus statement on the role of non-invasive testing from the Cardiac Imaging Committee, Council on Clinical Cardiology and the Cardiovascular Imaging and Intervention Committee, Council on Cardiovascular Radiology and Intervention of the AHA relates predominantly to women with an intermediate to high likelihood of CVD before testing [128]. The 2007 AHA guideline also recommended the **determination of women's CVD risk levels [129]. For both asymptomatic** and symptomatic women, initial test choice is guided by classifying women into low, intermediate, or high pre-test risk categories. Patients with diabetes and peripheral arterial disease are considered to be at high risk because both diabetes and peripheral arterial disease are considered CVD risk equivalents [128]. The pre-test likelihood of CVD, the characteristics of the baseline electro cardiogram, and the ability to exercise, are the major determinants choices for noninvasive tests [131].

Currently it seems that the exercise ECG was considered as the first line test for the evaluation of suspected cardiac symptoms in women [132]. American College of Cardiology/American Heart Association (ACC/AHA) exercise testing guidelines, suggested that women should undergo exercise testing if they are at an intermediate pre-test risk of CAD on the basis of symptoms and risk factors, have a normal resting ECG, and are capable of maximal exercise [132]. Both the diagnostic and prognostic accuracy of exercise electro cardiogram testing could be increased by inclusion of additional parameters, such as functional capacity and treadmill scores to the classic ST-segment response [131].

According to recent guidelines nonimaging exercise treadmill testing is useful for patients that have the ability to reach maximal level of exercise with a normal 12-lead resting ECG. But some factors may limit to achieve maximal exercise level in women. First, incidence of obesity and diabetes rapidly increase among women; these problems cause a decline in exercise capacity [128]. Secondly, menopausal status contributes a greater functional decline compared with similarly aged men and pre-menopausal women [133].

On the other hand, prevalence of non-obstructive CVD and single vessel disease is high among women. This factor induces to diminish diagnostic accuracy and higher false-positive rate for noninvasive testing in women versus men [128].

For women with an abnormal resting electrocardiogram, (i.e., resting ST-T wave changes that mask exercise-induced changes), and for women with indeterminate/ intermediate-risk exercise ECG results a cardiac imaging study is recommended. New techniques of echocardiography and radionuclide myocardial perfusion imaging enhanced the diagnostic and prognostic value of cardiovascular imaging in women with ischemic heart disease [134]. It was emphasized that stress echocardiography has greater diagnostic specificity and accuracy when compared with exercise electrocardiographic testing and it is valuable both for the recognition of CVD in women with chest pain syndromes and for their risk stratification [131].

Stress echocardiography with exercise or dobutamine can be used to detect the presence and location of wall motion abnormalities [134]. The rationale for its use is that cardiovascular stress will result in ischemia, which in turn is manifested as a regional wall motion abnormality distal to an obstructive coronary lesion [135]. This indicated that dobutamine stress echocardiography is an effective noninvasive tool in detecting CVD and assessing prognosis in women [136].

Pharmacologic stress testing is preferred for women who are unable to exercise to adequate intensity [131]. Pharmacologic stress myocardial perfusion imaging was used for diagnosis of known or suspected CVD in older women who have a decreased exercise capacity and in women who are not able to complete a symptom-limited exercise testing [137]. Also it is recommended for symptomatic women with normal or abnormal baseline ECG's who are not capable of maximal exercise [128].

Interventions of cardiac catheterization and coronary angiography were more often among men than women, but stress testing is applied more often in women. Even among the women who underwent coronary angiography, their testing was more delayed than was the case for men [131]. Existence of non-obstructive coronary artery disease in women with chest pain makes to establish diagnostic accuracy of coronary angiography difficult. One study has shown that at least 20% of women with normal or non-obstructive angiography have myocardial ischemia [75].

It was explained, some patients without angiographically detectable coronary stenoses, atherosclerosis may occur in a diffuse manner and lead to remodeling of the arterial wall, where the wall thickens and expands outward without encroaching on the lumen [138]. Also established, coronary macrovessel or microvessel dysfunction limits the coronary microcirculation during stress and therefore may be responsible for chest discomfort in the absence of obstructive CAD among women [139,140].

In 2006, the **Women's Ischemia Syndrome Evaluation** study received attention for the incorrect labeling of women with chest pain but without obstructive CVD as "low risk." It was determined that the future risk of adverse cardiovascular events such as MI was high in these patients [141].

Assessment of endothelial function should be recommended to determine the risk of future cardiac events in female patients with chest pain and normal or non-obstructive coronary angiograms [75, 141].

Endothelial dysfunction can hold the key for the early step in the development of atherosclerosis and it has been thought that its presence may be a determinant for an unfavorable cardiovascular prognosis [142]. Also reported, endothelial dysfunction is a reversible disorder; so traditional interventions for modifying cardiovascular risk factors, such as cholesterol lowering, smoking cessation, and contribute to improve endothelial function [142].

One study reported that women are less likely than men to receive angioplasty or an emergency bypass [143,144]. It was reported that gender specific physiological differences may affect treatment outcomes related to myocardial revascularization procedures and they were less favorable in women than in men [145]. Coronary vessels are smaller regardless of women's body size; so they are more prone to coronary occlusion compared to men. When revascularization is performed to reestablish blood flow to occluded arteries via percutaneous coronary intervention, or coronary artery bypass graft (CABG), the luminal diameter of an artery is a strong predictor of restenosis. In most balloon angioplasty series, women experienced higher complication and mortality rates [146]. The size of coronary vessel correlates with long term graft patency and may be associated with higher perioperative mortality rates in women after CABG [20, 147]. A recent study confirmed that female patients CABG have a higher incidence of adverse outcomes including death, which are not mitigated by careful matching with male patients [148].

Women with heart disease have greater morbidity and mortality and have lower physical and social functioning. CVD have clear negative effects on women's physical and emotional roles in the family life. It was observed, there was a decline in energy and activity levels and difficulties related performing household activities especially where it required upper-body movement, heavy lifting or pushing in women with heart disease [149,150]. Following these physical inabilities when coping with the CVD; it becomes increasing difficult among women, where psychological well being worsens and other problems such as lower self-esteem and feelings of guilt were seen in the women [151-154].

Compared to men, women with CVD have different behavioral and coping responses after acute cardiac events [108]. It has been found that social structural and psychosocial determinants of health generally tend to be more important for women's health, whereas behavioral determinants tend to be more important for men's health [155].

Loose and Fernhall's study shows women have significantly greater dysfunction in emotional behavior, home management, and psychosocial functioning; in spite of men having a higher functional capacity [156]. King's et al. study involved women who had undergone coronary bypass surgery. They evaluated optimism, coping strategies, and psychological and functional outcomes in women during hospitalization and at 1, 6, and 12 months postoperatively. Women reported the highest level of disruption in home management one month following surgery [157].

Further, illness and coping behaviors for a cardiac event are influenced by male and female gender roles [158]. It was established in this study that housekeeping facilitates increase ability of women to deal with the stress of illness [159]. When men have severe cardiac symptoms, they tend to assume less responsibility in partnership and household activities. But women with similar symptoms try to minimize the impact of their heart disease and to avoid burdening their social contacts [160]. Because of these differences in coping with heart disease between men and women; more supportive, more encouraging and more sensitive psychosocial interventions should be planned in female cardiac patients. According to literature, effective psychosocial interventions include elements of mediating knowledge, group support, and stress management [161,162]. Recently, Clark et al. research evaluated outcomes of different training formats in women with heart disease. The results of this research were interesting: self-directed women experienced improved outcomes over group women for symptoms, but group women did better regarding weight loss and ambulation [163].

Clinicians should experience different training alternatives for achieving good results in women with heart disease.

Chapter 5

DEPRESSION IN WOMEN WITH CVD

The screening and treatment of depression in women with overt CVD should not be ignored. Depression is a prevalent problem in most patients with heart disease [164].

Studies have indicated that after a cardiac event, depression is observed in 15 − 22% of patients and women are twice as likely to suffer from depression as men. Biologic factors such as fluctuating hormonal levels from menstrual cycle and reproduction, and some psychosocial factors may contribute to these gender differences. More atypical symptoms, anxiety and eating disorders, and longer and more recurrent depressive episodes were found in women with depression [165].

Major depression and depressive symptoms worsen prognosis and often reduces quality of life [166, 167]. Depression is associated with some physiologic changes, including nervous system activation, cardiac rhythm disturbances, systemic and localized inflammation, and hypercoagulability that negatively influence the cardiovascular system [168]. Additionally, depression is an important barrier to overcome when attempting to adopt healthier lifestyle behaviors to manage heart disease [169]. In patients who have CVD, depression is associated with a reduction in both short- and long-term survival [166, 170,171]. Barefoot *et al.* found that depressed individuals experienced a greater risk of mortality than did nondepressed individuals [171].

Etiological and prognostic studies indicate that depression may be a cause or a consequence of CVD [27]. Depression increases risk of adverse outcome after a diagnosis of heart disease [169]. One study related to depression following MI revealed an increased frequency of depression in women, with the greatest risk being reported in younger women [172]. This finding confirmed previous studies' opinion that there is a possibility of an association between depression and increased adverse outcomes in younger compared with older women following both MI and myocardial revascularization procedures [31, 173, 174]. Lack of social support/social integration, low socioeconomic status, vital exhaustion, and the presence of two or more depressive symptoms are considered as important predictors for recurrent cardiac events among women with heart disease [175, 176] Also it was indicated that after an acute myocardial infarction, women's psychosocial adjustment was worse than that of men [177]. On the other hand, women have specific apprehensions about emotional issues during their heart disease's recovery period. It was clearly demonstrated that women with heart disease need encouragement from others and peer support in this process. In this mean, group sessions may allow the sharing of knowledge and experiences and emotional support between group members [3, 178, 179].

It was indicated that women experience a poorer quality of life than men one year after acute MI [180]. Women have reported lower energy levels and more functional and psychosocial problems in quality of life subscales in other study [181, 182]. Major depression and depressive symptoms worsen prognosis and reduces quality of life [166, 167]. It is obvious that women with heart disease need professional psychosocial support. Women specific CVD management approaches may help to increase well-being in all areas of a women's life. Just as one randomized controlled trial suggested that a 1-year cognitive-behavioral stress management program designed specifically for women improved psychological well-being [183].

Some studies demonstrated that physical activity has a beneficial effect on psychological symptoms and psychiatric disorders [184]. This effect seems to be possible. First of all, during exercise, a woman spends this time specifically for herself. Although this exercise time is not long; she forgets personal and her family-related problems in this time. If women have a regular exercise habit, physically active life style can help cope with depression and promote psychological health.

GENERAL AIMS
OF CARDIAC REHABILITATION

Cardiac rehabilitation (CR) targets to optimize the physical, psychological, social functioning of patients and to reduce cardiovascular morbidity and mortality [184]. Purposes for achieving these goals are to help individuals to adapt to their illness, limit or reverse the disease, modify risk factors for future cardiac illness, improve return to occupational and social functioning, and reduce the risk of re-infarction or sudden death [185-187]. Internationally CR consists of three phases: (1) the inpatient phase; (2) the outpatient phase; and (3) the maintenance phase [188]. The initial phase begins in the hospital almost immediately following a MI or cardiac event. This phase of CR comprises patient education, basic daily activities such as sitting up in bed, joint range of motion techniques, and walking. Recently, a study by Evans *et al.* reported that the inpatient phase of CR should provide education and psychosocial support to the patients before dismissal from hospital. Instruction for patients should include the nature of the heart disease or intervention, and a cardiac risk factor assessment and modification [189].

The second phase is for early recovery, and consists of the first few weeks to months following the hospital stay. During this phase its focus targeted increase activity levels **according to patient's tolerance**, and start patient education related to lifestyle changes. The third phase objective is to give encouragement to patient to continue regular exercise habit. This phase is important for reducing the risk of additional cardiac events and associated mortality. Finally, the third phase is the maintenance that is recommended throughout the life of the patient [190].

Significant achievements have been obtained in CR. Many studies related to CR have been published in the literature and cardiac rehabilitation guidelines issued. Unfortunately, CR has tended to favor men [191].

Despite evidence that women are considered to be at high risk for recurrent coronary events and cardiac mortality [192]; female coronary patients have low referral and participation rates in CR programs [54, 193]. If women were elderly, obese, depressed, nonwhites, or those with greater comorbidity, lower exercise capacity, less social support, they were not incorporated into CR [194-196].

Previous studies demonstrated that adequate information increases the adherence to treatment programs and compliance to healthy life style behaviors [197,198].

Gender specific cardiac rehabilitation programs have remained somewhat limited [199]. Some guidelines mentioned women as a specific population [200 - 204]. Notably, a few gender-specific cardiac rehabilitation programs were initiated in recent years and these programs aimed at meeting women's need and preferences more efficiently than standard cardiac rehabilitation programs. Although existing gender-specific programs are similar to standard programs, they have women-specific goals which included positive self-concepts, assertiveness and the modification of unfavorable communication strategies [199].

Existence of women-specific guidelines is gratifying but they should be extended to include more content and become more prevalent. Another important point is to have these guidelines available to as many urban and rural women as possible. It is neccessary to provide easy understandable books to educate women, especially the young, to learn about the prevention of coronary heart disease. In this way, especially in developing countries; women's awareness level about protection against heart disease can be increased.

Chapter 7

COMPONENTS
OF CARDIAC REHABILITATION

Nowadays, one of the most important objectives of cardiac rehabilitation is minimizing the risk of further cardiac events. So, risk factor modification may be considered as milestone of CR for both prevention and management of CVD in healthy or ill individuals. In 2007, the American Heart Association (AHA) guideline for CVD prevention in women categorized the determination of women's CVD risk levels as high, intermediate, lower, and optimal risk. Classification was done according to clinical criteria and/or the Framingham global risk score. Women who have coronary heart disease, cerebrovascular disease, peripheral arterial disease, chronic renal disease, abdominal aortic aneurysm, diabetes mellitus, and >20% of 10-year Framingham global risk were in the high risk group. Women who have ≥1 major risk factors for CVD including cigarette smoking, poor diet, physical inactivity, obesity, family history of premature CVD, hypertension, dyslipidemia; evidence of subclinical vascular disease, metabolic syndrome, poor exercise capacity on treadmill test and/or abnormal heart rate recovery after stopping exercise were considered in the intermediate risk group. Women who have <10% of Framingham global risk and had a healthy lifestyle, with no risk factors; comprised as the optimal risk group [129]. Diabetes, dyslipidaemia, hypertension, smoking, obesity, sedentary lifestyle and poor nutrition are considered modifiable risk factors [129].

Primary and secondary prevention categories of the CR are based on the development or manifestation of atherosclerotic CVD. The new guideline also touches on the primary and secondary prevention of atherosclerotic vascular diseases. Both prevention efforts have similar strategies. They involve cardiovascular risk reduction, encourage healthy behavior and conformity with those behaviors and support an active lifestyle in patients with high-risk profile or CVD [117, 205].

Secondary prevention programs targeted to slow progression of CVD, enhance quality of life, and eventually reduce mortality in patients with known coronary artery disease [206].

The AHA 2007 guideline addresses issues related to lifestyle, risks to watch or avoid, and drugs to prevent heart disease. Lifestyle recommendations include avoid smoking, encouraging women to regular physical activity, adherence to a healthy eating pattern, weight maintenance/ reduction, and the use of omega-3 fatty acids. Major risk factor interventions are maintaining optimal blood pressure, lipid and lipoprotein levels and controlling diabetes mellitus. Preventive drug interventions are aspirin therapy, beta blockers, angiotensin converting enzyme inhibitor or angiotensin receptor blocker and aldosterone blockade [129, 207].

Regular exercise is a necessary component for a healthy lifestyle. Higher levels of exercise reduce both coronary risk factors (such as hypertension, obesity, diabetes) and risks of coronary heart disease [208]. A study reported that women who are sedentary are twice as likely to develop CVD compared to women who are not sedentary [209]. Yet, unfortunately statics have shown more than 60% of adult women fail to exercise to realize the health benefits [210].

Literature suggests that despite experiencing a recent life-threatening cardiac event and having attended a CR program, some women never exercised again; and only 50% were still exercising at the end of 3 months [211,212].

Although physical inactivity and poor nutrition are two of the most important modifiable risk factors for CVD in women, there are limited interventional studies for reducing these factors in women [213, 214].

Beckie's study denoted a disregard for women-oriented protocols. The study stated that although medically supervised exercise training is considered as the cornerstone of CR programs; treatment protocols have traditionally been based on a male model for medicine with women's health issues viewed as deviations from a male-defined norm [215].

Health-care providers should consider incentive programs to include different exercise alternatives that are beneficial for women. Many women may benefit from short counseling sessions during routine office visits, whereas others may need a more individualized exercise approach. Assist and support of a clinician is very helpful and useful for the transition into a more active and healthier lifestyle in women [1].

To provide CVD prevention and control strategies are more effective than individual strategies to achieve CR goals in women [129]. Pazoki *et al.* study had shown that a community-based study can be effective for the short term adoption of physical activity behavior among women [214].

Community-based CR programs should be increased and their outcomes should be assessed among women.

Chapter 8

BENEFITS OF CARDIAC
REHABILITATION IN WOMEN

When primary prevention efforts of CR for women were investigated; it is obvious that exercise have beneficial effects on CVD risk factors. Regular exercise improves blood lipid profile; leads to reduction in total cholesterol, in LDL-C and increase in HDL-C [216, 217]. Positive lipid effects of exercise may be more prominent in postmenopausal women than premenopausal women [216]. Additionally, regular physical activity increase exercise capacity, reduce angina symptoms and improve prognosis in cardiac patients [218,219]. It was demonstrated in postmenopausal women that moderate regular exercise reduced total mortality by 24-38% [220,221].

Exercise training helps to weight loss and the development of a more favorable body composition and fat distribution with regard to CVD risk [222]. Research shown that, physically active women have a more favorable waist-hip ratio than do sedentary women [223,224]. One lifestyle modification study done in Turkey had shown a reduction in hypertension and obesity ratio among women after training [225]. Studies have shown that regular physical activity is inversely associated with long-term cardiovascular mortality in both women and men [226-228]. A study that included postmenopausal women found that inverse relationship between leisure physical activity and cardiovascular mortality [220]. The success of the primary prevention programs for women may increase by determining the personal, psychological, and behavioral variables. After a regular participation in the prevention program, women transfer their knowledge about heart healthy behaviors to family members and/or other community members [229]. A recent systematic review exhibited that exercise-related improvement in body weight, bone constitution, muscle strength and endurance, flexibility, oxygen consumption, blood pressure, and metabolic control in women after menopause [230].

CR improves exercise tolerance, coronary risk factors, psychological well-being, and health-related quality of life in patients with heart disease [231-234]. Improvements regarding psychological well being included decreased levels of anxiety and depression, increase self-esteem, and better emotional and spiritual recovery [235].

Studies suggest that secondary prevention programs of CR also reduced long-term mortality [231- 234, 236]. One trial reported that mortality reduced by 20-25% after CR programs and these gains are similar in magnitude to those of major cardiac drugs and surgery [237].

The Cochrane Database on Exercise-Based Rehabilitation for Coronary Heart Disease concluded that exercise based cardiac rehabilitation effectively reduced cardiac death, without clear evidence as to whether an exercise-only or a comprehensive cardiac rehabilitation program   could be more beneficial. It was found that 27% reduction in total mortality after exercise- only based rehabilitation, but 13% reduction after comprehensive cardiac rehabilitation [238]. Evidence-based benefits of CR were summarized: an improvement in exercise tolerance, improvement in symptoms, improvement in blood lipid levels, reduction in cigarette smoking, improvement in psychosocial well-being, reduction of stress, and reduction in mortality, recurrent MI, and requirement for myocardial revascularization procedures [219, 239].

Do women benefit from CR programs devoted to secondary prevention as much as men do? The answer to this question is controversial because of limited data regarding exercise as secondary prevention in women. A recent systematic review and meta-analysis of randomized trials of exercise both alone and as a component of multidisciplinary CR involved women as one-fifth of the cohort and included a substantial representation of both patients > 65 years of age and those following myocardial revascularization procedures [219]. An early study by Oldridge and Bitner expressed that women and men may benefit equally from CR, with improvements in clinical, psychosocial, and behavioral outcomes [240, 241]. Ades et al. study found that there was no difference in improvement of peak aerobic capacity between males and females patients who enrolled CR program after MI and CABG [193]. Various studies on the gender-specific effectiveness of exercise exercise-based cardiac rehabilitation corroborated that women, achieved the same improvement in medical risk factors, functional capacity and quality of life [114, 182, 190, 242-245].

Two studies' had promising results for women. Savage's study documented that women experienced a significantly better improvement in HDL-C levels than men with CR [246]. More recently, Gupta's study suggested that women have better long-term retention and implementation of dietary advice and CR benefits remained significantly greater among women than among men one year later [247].

On the other hand, some previous results were not consistent with these mentioned findings. Two studies included women with coronary artery disease, showed no major effect on lipid values after CR [114, 190]. Allen examined risk factor management in women post CABG in his study. Results of the study demonstrated that one year later 58% remained obese, 54% continued to be hypertensive, and 92% continued to have elevated low-density lipoprotein cholesterol levels. These women sustained high risk profile [248]. Claesson et al. documented men have benefited much more than women from CR. In their study, the chance of long-term survival after a myocardial infarction doubled in men during a 10 year period from the mid-1980s, whereas no improvement at all was observed in women [236]. In another CR study that compared to women, men show greater improvements in some physical components such as body mass index [182].

Realization of health benefits is dependent on attendance and compliance to basic components of CR program (exercise training, diet etc.) Robiner emphasized continued attention to maximize adherence is important for enhancing treatment benefits [249]. Making instructions to subjects simpler and less demanding, addressing cognitive-motivational factors such as self-efficacy and health beliefs, offering social support and reinforcement, and providing reminders are some of developed strategies to promote adherence. Studies suggest that the highest success rates are achieved by a combination of this kind of personal approach [250, 251].

Understanding a patients' causal approach regarding coronary heart disease is another important issue in terms of witnessing effective gains in prevention programs. Previous studies have found that attendance rates for CR or lifestyle modification programs in patients who attribute their CVD to factors that may be outside their control, such as heredity and stress were low [252, 253].

Some studies suggest that the pattern of external attribution is more common among women than men [254-256]. It has been speculated that this difference may be a factor responsible for low attendance by women at CR programs [256].

Education for women with heart disease should also include accurate knowledge in the area of causal attributions and beliefs about their illness. Sharing information about successful outcomes in CR trials may be one of the helpful ways to encourage reluctant women to attend to CR programs.

Chapter 9

BARRIERS OF CARDIAC REHABILITATION IN WOMEN

Women typically have lower exercise capacity and lower exercise tolerance then men [257]. Parallel to these characteristics, other studies determined when after a cardiac event, it is difficult to motivate women than men to engage in regular physical activities [258, 259]. The research literature emphasized that women have a significantly lower rate of referral, are less likely to enroll and drop out before completing CR programs compared with their male counterparts. According to the research data: in the United States and Canada only approximately 25-31% of eligible patients do participate in CR programs, the rate for women being much lower at 11-20% of those eligible [260]. Similarly, some reports suggest a low level participation by women [261-263]. According to new studies, it unfortunately revealed no improvement in favor of women in recent years; participation rates among eligible women did not exceed 15% to 20%. [196, 264,265]

Research to explain possible causes of the sex disparity in CR utilization was examined. Previous reports [148, 266, 267] and recent studies [241, 268-270] addressed this particular issue. Identified determinants of CR participation were classified in three groups [271]: (1) patient-related factors, such as social support, family responsibilities, personal preferences, financial pressures, availability, ease of transportation, and severity of disease; (2) physician-related factors, such as the strength of the physician`s recommendation to patients for CR enrollment and the physician's perceptions regarding the benefits of CR for the patient; and (3) program-related factors, such as program costs, the desirability of class schedules and facilities, and program location/availability.

Studies over the past 10 years have shown that all the previously mentioned factors remained stable. According to the studies' results; most common barriers included advanced age, non-cardiac morbidity (such as diabetes, arthritis, and osteoporosis), high prevalence of depression and anxiety, less social support, inconvenient timings, and family responsibilities lessen the adherence rates in women [241, 268-270].

Age is the most consistent predictor regarding attendance to CR, with least attendance in younger (<49 years of age) and older (>70 years of age) women [193, 258, 271]. Some researchers have shown that younger age was an independent predictor of drop out but others reported the odds of completion doubled in patients less than 65 years of age [272-274]. Older women often suffer from co-morbid conditions such as arthritis, osteoporosis and urinary incontinence which lessen their motivation to physical activities [275, 276]. Also it has been reported that mobility problems and difficulties in using public transportation may limit the participation in outpatient, supervised, hospital-based CR of older individuals for whom home-based CR might be a valid alternative [257, 277]. At the same time, older women often are not accustomed to exercise at a high-intensity level and this negatively affects their participation and adherence to CR programs [278]. When planning CR programs for elderly women, perhaps age specific exercise limitations should be considered.

Worcester *et al.* reported the diabetes disease patients were associated with nonattendance amongst women, and according to their opinion these patients already had prescribed regimens for lifestyle change therefore did not recognize a need for an additional program of exercise and education [198].

Depression often makes adherence difficult when proscribing recommended changes in behavior and lifestyle [279-281]. It reduces the chances of successful modifications for other cardiac risk factors and participation in cardiac rehabilitation and exercise programs [280, 281]. Providing encouragement, follow-up contacts and family or partner's support may help to resolve adherence problems in depressive patients [282].

Women have more domestic tasks than men and generally women are primary caregiver for children [283-285]. Because of the general belief that care-giving is "women's work," women also undertake the role of care-giving for an elderly and/or ill person in the family [286]. It was stated that caregivers are less likely to have time to engage in self-care and preventive health behavior than woman who do not provide care [287]. It is well known today, that most women are professionally active [288,289]. When work related tasks were added to family responsibilities; more problems arise especially among white collar women [290-292]. Unfortunately, female patients may give priority to domestic and work related duties, at the expense of own their health. Based on observations from previous studies; women thought that attending CR would take time away from their partners, families, and friends and they were unable to attend these programs [286, 293].

Family encouragement for participation in CR is important to both men and women but encouragement from adult children is more important for women [241]. Women that do not get sufficient support from their families may refrain from becoming more physically active [294].

Race, education, socioeconomic status, and marital status are other demographic characteristics that affect compliance with CR. Lack of insurance and lower income limit enrollment [257, 295]. Previous studies found that there was a positive relationship between high education level and high attendance rate among women [241, 296-299]. Apple *et al* described women with low socio-economic status and educational level have difficulty adhering to a lifestyle modification program that consisted of balanced and optimal nutrition, physical exercise and healthy living [300]. It was also shown that there was a distinction in comparison to men, being married does not increase attendance at cardiac rehabilitation in women [219].

Environmental factors are important for identifying barriers concerning CR enrollment. They included accessibility of the program, practice norms and referral processes, and program attributes and services [301]. It was stated that geographical distance is common barrier to accessibility of CR programs for American women. When the location of CR center is too far from their home, attendance rates dropped off [257,258, 302-304]. Similarly, lack of transportation makes attending to CR difficult [293, 305]. It was shown that healthcare **professionals' encouragement** and cardiac surgical **team' referrals** are effective for regular attendance to CR programs in women [258, 305-307]. Consistent and encouraging feedback from CR program staff regarding progress is important to women [151, 308,309]. Also, previous studies suggest another important point is the overall harmony among the program's approach and **women's preferences for improve**ment in attendance. When the program did not provide coordination for their specific needs and expectations, women **refused the CR programs [293]. It was observed that women's levels of self-**efficacy with relation to exercise and tolerance levels for physical activity were lower than men's. **So women do not want** to exercise at a fatigue or pain level [310- 314]. Analogously, women do not prefer the predominant-male, gym-like atmosphere and the limited exercise options offered in most programs (treadmill and exercise bicycle) [309].

One recent study evaluated the reasons for withdrawal from CR programs in women compared with men. This study had shown that women were significantly more likely to withdraw from CRP than men because of greater medical problems, specifically musculoskeletal and multiple medical reasons. Also the study found lack of interest and work obligations were greater barriers for men while transportation and family obligations more often affected women [312].

When considered their multidimensional barriers to CR, women-oriented programs should be varied to allow a sensible type of program. Notably, the atmosphere and exercise options should be planned according to the preferences of women. For example, home-based CR programs may be a good alternative especially for older, or very busy women, or for women with social restrictions [313-315]. As a result, recommendations should be specific to each woman and her background. Also country-specific and cultural variations should be considered.

Chapter 10

FUTURE SUGGESTIONS FOR CARDIAC REHABILITATION IN WOMEN

The importance women have in the family and society is unchallenged, literality. Yet, unfortunately CVD continues to threaten women's lives. There is a need to develop effective interventions for increasing achievement and popularity of CR programs for women. It should be recognized that the flexibility of CR programs is more important for women than men. When research and studies on this issue were conducted about different physiological and clinical dimensions of women's CVD; women-specific psychological features, familial and social roles, needs, beliefs and expectations should be considered. It should be remembered that to protect women from heart disease is an important step for achieving a productive aging society.

REFERENCES

[1] Banks, AD. Women and heart disease: missed opportunities. *J Midwifery Womens Health* 53: 430-439,2008

[2] Starmba-Badiale, M; Fox, KM; Priori, SG., *et al.* Cardiovascular disease in women: a statement from the policy conference of the European Society of Cardiology. *Eur Heart J.* 27: 994-1005, 2006.

[3] Perry, CK., and Rosenfeld, AG. Learning through connections with others: women's cardiac symptoms. *Patient Educ Couns.* 57(1): 143-146, 2005.

[4] Mosca, L; Ferris, A; Fabunmi, R., *et al.* Tracking women's awareness of heart disease: An American Heart Association national study. *Circulation* 109: 573-579, 2004.

[5] American Heart Association Web site. Facts about women and cardiovascular diseases. Available at: *www.americanheart.org/presenter.jhtml?identifier=2876* Accessed August 8, 2006.

[6] Bello, N, and Mosca, L. Epidemiology of coronary heart disease in women. *Prog Cardiovasc Dis.* 46: 287-295, 2004.

[7] Petersen, S; Peto, V; Rayner, M; Leal, J; Luengo-Fernandez, R; and Gray, A. European cardiovascular disease statistics. Oxford: British Hearth Foundation, 2005. *www.heartstats.org/uploads/documents%5CPDF.pdf* (accessed 15 Aug 2005)

[8] National Institutes of Health, National Heart, Lung and Blood Institute. Heart disease deaths in American women decline. February 1, 2007. http: //www.nih.gov/news/pr/feb2007/nhlbi-01.htm. Accessed July 18, 2007.

[9]   Petersen, S; Peto, V; Scarborough, P; and Rayner, M. British Heart
      Foundation Health Promotion Research Group. Coronary heart disease
      statistics Oxford: British Hearth Foundation, 2005. *www.heartstats.*
      org/temp/CHD_2005_Whole_spdocument.pdf (accessed 15 Aug 2005)

[10] Yalçın, M, and Bardak, M. Health Statistics 1996. Republic of Turkey
      Ministry of Health, Research Planning and Coordination Committee.
      Ankara, 1970.

[11] Onat, A; Dursunoğlu, D; and Sansoy, V. Relatively high coronary death
      and event rates in Turkish women; Relation to three major risk factors in
      five year follow-up cohort. *Int J Cardiol.* 61: 69-77, 1997.

[12] New Zealand Health Information Statistics. May 7th, 2003. Mortality
      statistics: Totals for 1998 and 1999; (Website) New Zealand Health
      Information Services. Available:
      http://www.nzhis.govt.nz/stats/mortstats.html [2004, 12.5.04]

[13] Australian Institute of Health and Welfare. Australian Institute of Health
      and Welfare National Mortality Database. Department of Health and
      Human Services. Canberra, Australia: Australian Institute of Health and
      Welfare, 1999.

[14] Schenck-Gustafsson K. Risk factors for cardiovascular disease in
      women. Maturitas, 63: 186-190, 2009.

[15] Yusuf, S; Reddy, S; Ounpuu, S; and Anand, S. Global burden of
      cardiovascular diseases: part 1: general considerations, the
      epidemiologic transition, risk factors, and impact of urbanization.
      Circulation 104: 2746 –2753, 2001.

[16] Wizemann, TM, and Pardue, M-L (Eds); Committee on Understanding
      the Biology of Sex and Gender Differences, Board on Health Sciences
      Policy, Institute of Medicine (2001) Exploring the biological
      contributions to human health. Does sex matter? Washington: National
      Academy Press.

[17] Wenger, NK. You've come a long way, baby: cardiovascular health
      disease in women: problems and prospects. *Circulation* 109: 558–560,
      2004.

[18] Anand, SS; Islam, S; Rosengren, A; *et al.* Investigators risk factors of
      myocardial infarction in women and men: insights from the
      INTERHEART study. *Eur Heart J.* 29(7): 937-952, 2008.

[19] Legato, MJ. Gender-specific physiology: how real is it? How important
      is it? *Int J Fertil.* 42:19-29, 1997.

[20] Shefier, S; Canos, M; Weinfurt, K; *et al.* Sex differences in coronary artery size assessed by intravascular ultrasound. *Am Heart J.* 139: 649-653, 2000.

[21] Mosca, L; Manson, JE; Sutherland, SE; *et al.* Cardiovascular disease in women: A statement for healthcare professionals from the American Heart Association Writing Group. *Circulation* 96: 2468-2482, 1997

[22] Mosca, L; Novel cardiovascular risk factors: Do they add value to your practice? *Am Family Physician* 67: 264, 2003.

[23] Pepys, MB, and Hirschfield, GM. C-reactive protein. *J Clin Invest.* 111 (12): 1805–1812, 2003. doi: 10.1172/JCI18921

[24] Ridker, PM; Cushman, M; Stampfer, MJ; *et al.* Inflammation, aspirin, and the risk of cardiovascular disease in apparently healthy men. *N Engl J Med.* 336: 973–979, 1997.

[25] Ridker, PM; Buring, JE; Shih, J; *et al.* Prospective study of C-reactive protein and the risk of future cardiovascular events among apparently healthy women. *Circulation* 98: 731-733, 1998.

[26] Bittner, V. State of the art paper: perspectives on dyslipidemia and coronary heart disease in women. *J Am Coll Cardiol.* 46:1628– 1635, 2005.

[27] Möller-Leihmkühler, AM. Women with coronary artery disease and depression: A neglected risk group. *The World J Biol Psychiatry*, 9(2): 92-101, 2008.

[28] Ades, P; Tischler, MD; Savage, PD; *et al.* Determinants of disability in older coronary patients. *Circulation* 94 (Suppl 1): (I-497), 1996.

[29] Eastwood, JA, and Doering, LV. Gender differences in coronary artery disease. *J Cardiovasc Nurs.* 20: 340-351, 2005.

[30] National Heart, Lung, and Blood Institute. The healthy heart handbook for women. NIH, 2007.

[31] Vaccarino, V; Parsons, L; Every, NR; *et al.* Sex-based differences in early mortality after myocardial infarction. *New Engl J Med.* 41:217-225, 1999.

[32] Van der Giezen, AM; Schopman-Geurts van Kessel, JG; Schouten, EG; *et al.* Systolic blood pressure and cardiovascular mortality among 13,740 Dutch women. *Prev Med.* 19: 456-465, 1990.

[33] Executive Summary. Women and smoking: A report of the Surgeon General. Morbid *Mortal Wkly Rep.* 51: 1-30, 2002.

[34] Limacher, MC. Coronary heart disease in women: past gaps, present state and future promises. *J Fla Med Assoc.* 83 (7):455-458, 1996.

[35] Jadin, RL, and Margolis, K. Coronary artery disease in women: how customary expectations can interfere with interpretation of test results. *Postgrad Med.* 103 (3): 71-84, 1998.

[36] Douglas, PS, and Ginsburg, GS. The evaluation of chest pain in women. *N Engl J Med.* 334 (20):1311-1315, 1996.

[37] Willett, WC; Green, A; Stampfer, MJ; *et al.* Relative and absolute excess risks of coronary heart disease among women who smoke cigarettes. *N Engl J Med.* 317: 1303- 1309, 1987.

[38] Cullen, P; Schulte, H; and Assmann, G. Smoking, lipoproteins and coronary heart disease risk. *Eur Heart J.* 19: 1632-1641, 1998.

[39] Castelli, WP. Cardiovascular disease: pathogenesis, epidemiology, and risk among users of oral contraceptives who smoke. *Am J Obstet Gynecol.* 180: 349-356, 1999.

[40] Polk, ND, and Naqvi, TZ. Cardiovascular disease in women: sex differences in presentation, risk factors, and evaluation. *Curr Cardiol Rep.* 7: 166-172, 2005.

[41] Toth, PP. The "Good Cholesterol": High-density lipoprotein *Circulation.* 111: 89-91, 2005.

[42] Triglycerides, High-Density Lipoprotein, and Coronary Heart Disease. *NIH Consensus Statement.* Vol. 10. No. 2. Bethesda, Md: Office of Medical Applications Research, 1992.

[43] Boden, WE. High-density lipoprotein cholesterol as an independent risk factor in cardiovascular disease: assessing the data from Framingham to the Veterans Affairs High-Density Lipoprotein Intervention Trial. *Am J Cardiol.* 86(12A):19L-22L, 2000.

[44] National Institute of Health. Third Report of the National Cholesterol Education Program Expert Panel on Detection, Evaluation, and Treatment of High Blood Cholesterol in Adults (ATP III). Bethesda, Md: NIH; 2001. Publication no. 0- 3670.

[45] Arnett, DK, and Province, MA; Investigators of the NHLBI family heart study. Lifestyle determinants of high-density lipoprotein cholesterol: the National Heart, Lung, and Blood Institute Family Heart Study. *Am Heart J.* 147: 529–535, 2004.

[46] Gordon, DJ; Probstfield, JL; Garrison, RJ; *et al.* High-density lipoprotein cholesterol and cardiovascular disease: four prospective American studies. *Circulation* 79: 8-15, 1989.

[47] Skoumas, J; Pitsavos, C; Panagiotakos, DB; Chrysohoou, C; Zeimbekis, A; Papaioannou, I; Toutouza, M; Toutouza, P; and Stefanadis, C. Physical activity, high density lipoprotein cholesterol and other lipids

levels, in men and women from the ATTICA study. *Lipids Health Disease* 2: 3-10, 2003.

[48] Dorn, JM; Schistermann, EF; Winkelstein, W; *et al.* Body mass index and mortality in a general population sample of men and women: The Buffalo Health Study. *Am J Epidemiol.* 1146: 919-931, 1997.

[49] Kenachaiah, S; Gaziano, JM, and Vasan, RS. Impact of obesity on the risk of heart failure and survival after the onset of heart failure. *Med Clin N Am.* 88:1273-1294, 2004.

[50] Garrison, RJ; Higgins, MW; and Kannel, WB. Obesity and coronary heart disease. *Curr Opin Lipidol.* 7: 199-202, 1996.

[51] Anderson, J, and Kessenich, CR. Women and Coronary Heart Disease *Nurse Pract.* 26(8): 12-31, 2001.

[52] Chasan-Taber, L, and Stampfer, MJ. Epidemiology of oral contraceptives and cardiovascular disease. *Ann Intern Med.*128: 467-477, 1998.

[53] Grodstein, F; Manson, JE; and Stampfer, MJ. Postmenopausal hormone use and secondary prevention of coronary events in the Nurses' Health Study. *Ann Intern Med.* 135 (1): 1-8, 2001.

[54] Thomas, RJ; Houston-Miller, N; Lamendola, C; *et al.* National survey on gender differences in cardiac rehabilitation programs. *J Cardiopulm Rehabil.* 16: 402-412, 1996.

[55] Cannistra, LB; O'Malley, CJ; Balady, GJ. Comparison of outcome of cardiac rehabilitation in black women and white women. *Am J Cardiol.* 75: 890-893, 1995.

[56] Onat, A; Şurdum–Avcı, G; Şenocak, M ; *et al.* Screening of heart diseases and risk factors frequency in Turkey. Third prevalence of heart diseases. *Turkish Cardiol Assoc Arch* 19: 26-33, 1991. (Turkish).

[57] Kazemy, T, and Sharifzadeh, GR. Sex differences in acute myocardial infarction in Birjand Eastern Iran. *ARYA J.* 3(1): 42-44, 2007.

[58] Sasaki, J; Kita, T; Mabuchi, H ; *et al.* Gender difference in coronary events in relation to risk factors in Japanese hypercholesterolemic patients treated with low-dose simvastatin. *Circul J.*70: 810–814, 2007.

[59] Gu, D ; Gupta, A ; Muntner, P ; *et al.* Prevalence of cardiovascular disease risk factor clustering among the adult population of China: SHEEP Study Group. Stockholm Heart Epidemiology Program. *Am J Public Hlth.* 88: 382–388, 1998.

[60] Wamala, SP ; Murray, MA ; Horsten, M ; *et al.* Socioeconomic status and determinants of haemostatic function in healthy women. *Arterioscler Thromb Vasc Biol.* 19: 485–492, 1999.

[61] Knox, SS, and Follmann, D. Gender differences in the psychosocial variance of Framingham and Bortner Type A measures. *J Psychosom Res.* 37: 709-716, 1993.

[62] Friedman, M; Thoresen, CE; Gill, JJ; *et al.* Alteration of type A behavior and its effect on cardiac recurrences in post myocardial infarction patients: summary results of the recurrent coronary prevention project. *Am Heart J.* 112: 653–665, 1986.

[63] Eaker, ED. Psychosocial factors in the epidemiology of coronary heart disease in women. *Psychiatr Clin North Am.* 12:167-173, 1989.

[64] Hall, EM; Johnson, JV; and Tsou, T. Women, occupation, and risk of cardiovascular morbidity and mortality. *Occup Med.* 8: 709–719, 1993.

[65] Wamala, SP. Large social inequalities behind women's risk of coronary disease. Unskilled work and family strains are crucial factors (in Swedish). *Swedish Med J.* 98: 177–181, 2001.

[66] Orth-Gomer, K; Wamala, SP; Horsten, M; *et al.* Marital stress worsens prognosis in women with coronary heart disease: the Stockholm Female Coronary Risk Study. *JAMA.* 284: 3008–3014, 2000.

[67] Blom, M; Janszky, I; Balog, P; *et al.* Social relations in women with coronary heart disease: the effects of work and marital stres. *J Cardiovasc Risk* 10: 201–206, 2003.

[68] Hallman, T; Burell, G; Setterlind, S; *et al.* Psychosocial risk factors for coronary heart disease, their importance compared with other risk factors and gender differences in sensitivity. *J Cardiovasc Risk* 8 (1): 39- 49, 2001.

[69] Beckie, TM; Fletcher, GF; Beckstead, JW; *et al.* Adverse baseline physiological and psychosocial profiles of women enrolled in a cardiac rehabilitation clinical trial. *J Cardiopul Rehabil & Prev.* 28: 52–60, 2008.

[70] Perkins-Porras, L; Whitehead, DL, and Steptoe, A. Patients' beliefs about the causes of heart disease: relationships with risk factors, sex and socio-economic status. *Eur J Cardiovasc Prev Rehab* 13: 724–730, 2006.

[71] Nelson, HD. Menopause. *Lancet* 371: 760–770, 2008.

[72] Stevenson, JC. HRT and cardiovascular disease. *Best Practice & Res Clin Obstetrics & Gynaecol* 23: 109-120, 2009.

[73] Unal, B; Critchley, JA, and Capewell, S. Explaining the decline in coronary heart disease mortality in England and Wales between 1981 and 2000. *Circulation* 109:1101–1107, 2004.

[74] Bugiardini, R, and Bairey-Merz, CN. Angina with "normal" coronary arteries: a changing philosophy. *JAMA* 293: 477–484, 2005.

[75] Jacobsen, BK; Nilssen, S; Heuch, I; *et al.* Does age at natural menopause affect mortality from ischemic heart disease? *J Clin Epidemiol.* 50(4): 475-479, 1997.

[76] Gold, EB; Bromberger, J; Crawford, S; *et al.* Factors associated with age at natural menopause in a multiethnic sample of midlife women. *Am J Epidemiol.* 153: 865–874, 2001.

[77] Cramer, DW, and Xu, H. Predicting age at menopause. *Maturitas* 23: 319–326, 1996.

[78] Kato, I; Toniolo, P; Akhmedkhanov, A; *et al.* Prospective study of factors influencing the onset of natural menopause. *J Clin Epidemiol.* 51(12):1271-1276, 1998.

[79] Cramer, DW; Harlow, BL; Xu, H; *et al.* Cross-sectional and case-controlled analyses of the association between smoking and early menopause. *Maturitas* 22(2):79-87, 1995.

[80] Cooper, GS; Sandler, DP, and Bohlig, M. Active and passive smoking and the occurrence of natural menopause. *Epidemiol.* 10(6): 771-773, 1999.

[81] Mikkelsen, TF; Graff-Iversen, S; Sundby, J; *et al.* Early menopause, association with tobacco smoking, coffee consumption and other lifestyle factors: a cross-sectional study. *BMC Public Health* 7: 149-157, 2007.

[82] Luborsky, JL; Meyer, P; Sowers, MF; *et al.* Premature menopausein a multi-ethnic population study of the menopause transition. *Hum Reprod.* 18: 199–206, 2003.

[83] Stanford, JL; Hartge, P; Brinton, LA; *et al.* Factors influencing the age at natural menopause. *J Chronic Dis.* 40: 995–1002, 1987.

[84] Parazzini, F; Negri, E, and La Vecchia, C. Reproductive and general lifestyle determinants of age at menopause. *Maturitas* 15: 141– 149, 1992.

[85] Sievert, LL; Waddle, D, and Canali, K. Marital status and age at natural menopause: considering pheromonal influence. *Am J Human Biol.* 13: 479–485, 2001.

[86] Colditz, GA; Willett, WC; Stampfer, MJ; *et al.* Menopause and the risk of coronary heart disease in women. *N Engl J Med.* 316:1105–1110, 1987.

[87] Kok, HS; van Asselt, KM; van der Schouv, YT; *et al.* Heart disease risk determines menopausal age rather than the reverse. *J Am Coll Cardiol.* 47: 1976-1983, 2006.

[88] Stevenson, JC; Crook, D, and Godsland, IF. Influence of age and menopause on serum lipids and lipoproteins in healthy women. *Atherosclerosis* 98: 83-90, 1993.

[89] Napoli, C; Williams-Ignarro, S; Nigris, F; *et al.* Physical training and metabolic supplementation reduce spontaneous atherosclerotic plaque rupture and prolong survival in hypercholesterolemic mice. *PNAS* 103: 10479–10484, 2006.

[90] Proudler, AJ; Felton, CV, and Stevenson, JC. Aging and the response of plasma insulin, glucose and C-peptide concentrations to intravenous glucose in postmenopausal women. *Clin Sci.* 83: 489-494, 1992.

[91] Ley, CJ; Lees, B, and Stevenson, JC. Sex and menopause-associated changes in body-fat distribution. *Am J Clin Nutr.* 55: 950-954, 1992.

[92] Poehlman, ET; Toth, MJ, and Gardner, AW. Changes in energy balance and body composition at menopause: A controlled, longitudinal study. *Ann Intern Med.* 123: 673-675, 1995.

[93] Winkler, UH. Menopause, hormone replacement therapy and cardiovascular disease: a review of haemostaseological findings. *Fibrinolysis* 6(Suppl 3): 5-10, 1992.

[94] Wiinber, N; Hoegholm, A; Christensen, HR; *et al.* 24-h ambulatory blood pressure in 352 normal Danish subjects, related to age and gender. *Am J Hypertens.* 8: 978–986, 1995.

[95] Mercuro, G ; Saiu, F ; Deidda, M ; *et al.* Impairment of physical exercise capacity in healthy postmenopausal women. *Am Heart J.* 151: 923– 927, 2006.

[96] Mercuro, G ; Longu, G ; Zoncu, S ; *et al.* Impaired forearm blood flow and vasodilator reserve in healthy postmenopausal women. *Am Heart J.* 137: 692– 697, 1999.

[97] Herrington, DM; Braden, GA; Williams, JK; *et al.* Endothelial-dependent coronary vasomotor responsiveness in postmenopausal women with and without estrogen replacement therapy. *Am J Cardiol.* 73: 951–952, 1994.

[98] Yoshioka, J; Node, K; Hasegawa, S; *et al.* Impaired cardiac response to exercise in postmenopausal women: relationship with peripheral vascular function. *Nucl Med Commun.* 24: 383–389, 2003.

[99] Mercuro, G ; Saiu, F ; Deidda, M ; *et al.* Effect of Hormone Therapy on Exercise Capacity in Early Postmenopausal Women. *Obstet Gynecol.* 110: 780–787, 2007.

[100] Avis, NE ; Brambilla, D ; McKinlay, SM ; *et al.* A longitudinal analysis of the association between menopause and depression: results from the Massachusetts women's health survey. *Ann Epidemiol.* 4: 212-214, 1994.

[101] Cruz, I; Serna, C, and Real, J. Ischemic heart disease and primary care: identifying gender-related differences. An observational study. *BMC Family Practice* 9: 60, 2008. doi:10.1186/1471-2296-9-60.

[102] Nilsson, P; Brandstrom, H; Lingfors, H; *et al.* Gender differences in secondary prevention of coronary heart disease: reasons to worry or not? (Quality assurance of secondary prevention of coronary artery disease. Ongoing project offers possibilities for improved treatment.) *Scand J Prim Health Care* 21: 37-42, 2003.

[103] Verbruggei, LM. Sex differentials in health. *Prevention* 97: 417- 437, 1982.

[104] Perry, CK, and Rosenfeld, AG. Learning through connections with others: women's cardiac symptoms. *Patient Educ Couns.* 57(1): 143-146, 2005.

[105] Vaccarino, V; Krumholz, HM, and Yarzebski, J. Sex differences in 2-year mortality after hospital discharge for myocardial infarction. *Ann Intern Med.* 134:173–181, 2001.

[106] Karcioglu, O; Unal-Aslan, B, and Aslan, O. Gender differences in the management and survival of patients with acute myocardial infarction. *Eur J Intern Med.* 13: 474-479, 2002.

[107] Riegel, B, and Gocka, I. Gender differences in adjustment to acute myocardial infarction. *Heart Lung* 24: 457–466, 1995.

[108] Simon, T; Mary-Krause, M; Cambou, JP; *et al.* USIC Investigators. Impact of age and gender on in-hospital and late mortality after acute myocardial infarction: increased early risk in younger women: results from the French nation-wide USIC registries. *Eur Heart J.* 27: 1282–1288, 2006.

[109] Stramba-Badiale, M; Fox, KM; Priori, SG ; *et al.* Cardiovascular disease in women: a statement from the policy conference of the European Society of Cardiology. *Eur Heart J.* 27: 994-1005 2006.

[110] Wenger, NK. Coronary heart disease: The female heart is vulnerable. *Prog Cardiovasc Disease* 46: 199-229, 2003.

[111] Mikhail, GW. Coronary heart disease in women. *BMJ* 331: 467, 2005

[112] Tofler, GH; Stone, PH, and Muller, JE. Effects of gender and race on prognosis after myocardial infarction: adverse prognosis for women, particularly black women. *J Am Coll Cardiol.* 83: 484-491, 1987.

[113] Cannistra, LB; Balady, GJ; O'Malley, CJ; *et al.* Comparison of the clinical profile and outcome of women and men in cardiac rehabilitation. *Am J Cardiol.* 69: 1274-1279, 1992.

[114] Sullivan, AK; Holdright, DR; Wright, CA; *et al.* Chest pain in women: clinical, investigative, and prognostic features. *BMJ* 308: 883– 886, 1994.

[115] Pope, J; Aufderheide, T; Ruthazer, R; *et al.* Missed diagnoses of acute cardiac ischemia in the emergency department. *N Engl J Med.* 342:1163-1170, 2000.

[116] Guidelines for Cardiac Rehabilitation and Secondary Prevention Programs / American Association of Cardiovascular and Pulmonary Rehabilitation Human Kinetics, pp. 139-142, 1999.

[117] McSweeney, JC; Marisue, C; O'Sullivan, P; *et al.* Women's early warning symptoms of acute myocardial infarction. *Circulation* 108: 2619-2123, 2003.

[118] Shephard, R, and Franklin, B. Changes in the quality of life: A major goal of cardiac rehabilitation. *J Cardiopulm Rehabil.* 21: 189, 2001.

[119] Murabito, JM. Women and cardiovascular disease: Contributions from the Framingham heart study. *J Am Med Womens Assoc.* 50:35-40, 1995.

[120] Wenger, N. Preventing cardiovascular disease in women: an update. *Clin Cardiol.* 31: 109-113, 2008.

[121] King, KM, and Collins-Nakai, RL. Short term recovery from cardiac surgery in women; suggestions for practice. *Can J Cardiol.* 14: 1367-1371, 1998.

[122] King, KM, and Gortner, SR. Women's short term recovery from cardiac surgery. *Prog Cardiovasc Nurs.* 11: 5-15, 1996.

[123] Meisler, JG. Toward optimal health: the experts discuss heart disease in women. *J Womens Health Gend Based MED* 10: 17-25, 2001.

[124] Marrugat, J; Sala, J. and Aboal, J. Epidemiology of cardiovascular disease. *Rev Esp Cardiol* 59(39): 264-274, 2006.

[125] Alter, DA; Naylor, CD, and Austin, PC. Biology or bias: practice patterns and long-term outcomes for men and women with acute myocardial infarction, *J Am Coll Cardiol.* 39: 1909–1916, 2002.

[126] Grady, D; Chaput, L, and Kristof, M. Results of systematic review of research on diagnosis and treatment of coronary heart disease in women. Evidence report/technology assessment No. 80. Rockville, MD: Agency

for Healthcare Research and Quality; May 2003. AHRQ Publication No. 03-0035.

[127] Mieres, JH; Shaw, LJ; Arai, A ; *et al.* Role of noninvasive testing in the clinical evaluation of women with suspected coronary artery disease: consensus statement from the Cardiac Imaging Committee, Council on Clinical Cardiology, and the Cardiovascular Imaging and Intervention Committee, Council on Cardiovascular Radiology and Intervention, American Heart Association. *Circulation* 111: 682–696, 2005.

[128] Mosca, L; Banka, CL; Benjamin, EJ; *et al.* Evidence based guidelines for cardiovascular disease prevention in women 2007 update. *Circulation* 115: 1481-1501, 2007.

[129] Mosca, L; Grundy, SM, and Judelson, D. Guide to preventive cardiology for women: AHA/ACC Scientific Statement: consensus panel statement. *Circulation.* 99: 2480–2484, 1999.

[130] Wenger, NK. Coronary heart disease in women: highlights of the past 2 years—stepping stones, milestones and obstructing boulders. *Nat Clin Pract Cardiovasc Med.* 3(4): 194-202, 2006.

[131] Gibbons, RJ; Balady, GJ; Bricker, JT ; *et al.* American College of Cardiology/American Heart Association Task Force on Practice Guidelines (Committee to Update the 1997 Exercise Testing Guidelines). *Circulation* 106: 1883–1892, 2002.

[132] Rosamond, W; Flegal, K; Friday, G; *et al.* Heart disease and stroke statistics—2007 update: a report from the American Heart Association Statistics Committee and Stroke Statistics Subcommittee. *Circulation* 115: 69–171, 2007

[133] Makaryus, AN; Shaw, LJ, and Mieres, JH. Diagnostic strategies for heart disease in women an update on imaging techniques for optimal management *Cardiology in Review* 15: 279–287, 2007.

[134] Armstrong, WF, and Zoghbi, WA, Stress Echocardiography current methodology and clinical applications *J Am Coll Cardiol.* 45: 1739–1747, 2005.

[135] Cortigiani, L ; Dodi, C ; Paolini, EA ; *et al.* Prognostic value of pharmacological stress echocardiography in women with chest pain and unknown coronary artery disease. *J Am Coll Cardiol.* 32:1975–1981, 1998.

[136] results from the International Collaborative Study of Cardiovascular Disease in Asia (InterAsia). *Circulation* 112: 658–665, 2005.

[137] Theorell, T; Tsutsumi, A; Hallquist, J; *et al.* Decision latitude, job strain, and myocardial infarction: a study of working men in Stockholm. The

[138] Klocke ,FJ; Baird, MG; Lorell, BH; *et al.* ACC/AHA/ASNC guidelines for the clinical use of cardiac radionuclide imaging—executive summary: a report of the American College of Cardiology/American Heart Association Task Force on Practice Guidelines (ACC/AHA/ASNC Committee to revise the 1995 guidelines for the clinical use of cardiac radionuclide imaging). *Circulation* 108: 1404–1418, 2003.

[139] Schoenhagen, P; Nissen, SE, and Tuzcu, EM. Coronary arterial remodeling: from bench to bedside. *Curr Atheroscler Rep.* 5:150-154, 2003.

[140] Camici, PG ; Marraccini, P ; Lorenzoni, R ; *et al.* Coronary hemo dynamics and myocardial metabolism in patients with syndrome X: response to pacing stress. *J Am Coll Cardiol.*17:1461–1470, 1991.

[141] Johnson, BD; Shaw, LJ; Pepine, CJ; *et al.* Persistent chest pain predicts cardiovascular events in women without obstructive coronary artery disease: results from the NIH-NHLBI-sponsored Women's Ischemia Syndrome Evaluation (WISE) study *Eur Heart J.* 27: 1408– 1415, 2006.

[142] Shaw, LJ; Bairey-Merz, CN; Pepine, CJ; *et al.* Insights from the NHLBI sponsored Women's Ischemia Syndrome Evaluation (WISE) study, Part 1: gender differences in traditional and novel risk factors, symptom evaluation, and gender-optimized diagnostic strategies. *J Am Coll Cardiol.* 47(3 Suppl): S4– S20, 2006.

[143] Bonetti, PO; Lerman, LO, and Lerman, A. Endothelial dysfunction: a marker of atherosclerotic risk. *Arterioscler. Thromb. Vasc. Biol.* 23; 168-175, 2003.

[144] Bellasi, A; Raggi, P; Bairey-Merz, CN; *et al.* New insights into ischemic heart disease in women. *Cleve Clin J Med.* 74(8): 585-594, 2007.

[145] Anand, SS; Xie, CC; Mehta, S; *et al.* Differences in the management and prognosis of women and men who suffer from acute coronary syndromes. *J Am Coll Cardiol* 2005; 46: 1845-1851.

[146] Jacobs, AK; Johnston, JM; Haviland, A; *et al.* Improved outcomes for women undergoing contemporary percutaneous coronary intervention: a report from the National Heart, Lung, and Blood Institute Dynamic registry. *J Am Coll Cardiol.* 39:1608–1614, 2002.

[147] Kelsey, SF; James, M; Holubkov, AL; *et al.* Results of percutaneous transluminal coronary angioplasty in women. 1985-1986 National Heart, Lung, and Blood Institute's Coronary Angioplasty Registry. *Circulation* 87: 720-727, 1993.

[148] O'Connor, M, and Morton, J. Effect of coronary artery diameter in patients undergoing coronary bypass surgery. *Circulation* 93: 652-655, 1996.

[149] Kasirajan, V; Wolfe, LG, and Medina, A. Institutional report – Coronary adverse influence of female gender on outcomes after coronary bypass surgery: a propensity matched analysis. *Interact Cardio Vasc Thorac Surg.* 8: 408–411, 2009.

[150] Kimble, LP. Impact of cardiac symptoms on self reported household task performance in women with coronary artery disease. *J Cardiopulm Rehabil.* 21: 18-23, 2001.

[151] Wilke, NA; Sheldahl, L, and Dougherty, S. Energy expenditure during household tasks in women with coronary artery disease. *Am J Cardiol* 75: 670-674, 1995.

[152] Moore, S, and Kramer, FM. Women's views of cardiac rehabilitation programs. *J Cardiopulm Rehabil.* 16: 163-168, 1996.

[153] Charity, LA. The experiences of postmenopausal women with coronary artery disease. *West J Nurs Res.* 19: 583-607, 1997.

[154] Charity, LA. The experiences of younger women with coronary artery disease. *J Womens Health Gend Based Med.* 8: 773-785, 1999.

[155] Hawthorne, MH. Gender differences in recovery after coronary artery surgery. *Image J Nurs Scholarsh.* 26: 75-80, 1994.

[156] Denton, M; Prus, S, and Walters, V. Gender differences in health: a Canadian study of the psychosocial, structural and behavioral determinants of health. *Soc Sci Med.* 58: 2585-2600, 2004.

[157] Loose, M., and Fernhall, B. Differences in quality of life among male and female cardiac rehabilitation participants. *J Cardiopulm Rehabil.* 15(3), 225-231, 1995.

[158] King, KB, Rowe, MA; Kimble, LP, and Zerwic, JJ. Optimism, coping and long-term recovery from coronary artery surgery in women. *Res Nurs Hlth*, 21: 15-26, 1998.

[159] Lemos, K; Suls, J; Jenson, M ; *et al.* How do female and male cardiac patients and their spouses share responsibilities after discharge from the hospital? *Ann Behav Med.* 25: 8-15, 2003.

[160] Kristofferzon, ML; Lofmark, R, and Carlsson, M. Myocardial infarction: gender differences in coping and social support. *J Adv Nurs.* 44: 360-374, 2003.

[161] Mittag, O; Horres-Sieben, B, and Maurischat, C. Psychological status and coping precess following ischemic heart disease: the role of age and gender. *Herzmedizin* 23: 70-76, 2006.

[162] Nunes, EV; Frank, KA, and Kornfeld, DS. Psychologic treatment for the type A behavior pattern and for coronary heart disease: a meta analysis of the literature. *Psychosom Med.* 49: 159-173, 1987.

[163] Burell, G. and Granlund, B. Women's hearts need special treatment. *Int J Behav Med.* 9(3): 228-242, 2002.

[164] Clark, NM; Janz, NK; Dodge, JA; Lin, X; Trabert, BL; Kaciroti, N; Mosca, L; Wheeler, JR, and Keteyian, S. Heart disease management by women: does intervention format matter? *Hlth Educ Behav.* 36; 394-409, 2009.

[165] Ahto, M; Isoaho, R; Puolijoki, H; et al. Coronary heart disease and depression in the elderly: a population based study. *Family Pract.* 14: 436-445, 1997.

[166] Kessler, RC; McGonagle, KA; Swartz, M; et al. Sex and depression in the National Comorbidity Survey, 1: life time prevalence, chronicity and recurrence. *J Affect Disord.* 29: 85–96, 1993.

[167] Benz-Scott, LA; Benor, K, and Allen, JK. Why are women missing form outpatient cardiac rehabilitation programs? A review of multilevel factors affecting referral, enrolment and completion. *J Womens Hlth* 11: 773-791, 2002.

[168] Orth-Gomer, K. Psychosocial and behavioral aspects of cardiovascular disease prevention in men and women. *Curr Opin Psychiatry* 20: 147-151, 2007.

[169] Miller, TQ; Smith, TW; Turner, CW; et al. A meta-analytic review of research on hostility and physical health. *Psychol Bull* 119: 322-348, 1996.

[170] Glassman, AH; O'Connor, CM; Califf, RM; et al. For the Sertraline Antidepressant Heart Attack Randomized Trial (SADHHEART) Group. Sertraline treatment of major depression in patients with acute MI or unstable angina *JAMA* 288: 701-709, 2002.

[171] Hance, M; Carney, RM; Freedland, KE; et al. Depression in patients with coronary heart disease: a 12-month follow-up. *Gen Hosp Psychiatry* 18: 61-65, 1996.

[172] Barefoot, JC; Helms. MJ; Mark, DB, et al. Depression and long-term mortality risk in patients with coronary artery disease. *Am J Cardiol.* 78:613-617, 1996.

[173] Mallik, S; Spertus, JA; Reid, KJ; et al. Depressive symptoms after acute myocardial infarction evidence for highest rates in younger women *Arch Intern Med.* 166: 876-883, 2006.

[174] Vaccarino, V; Abramson, JL; Emir, V ; *et al.* Sex differences in hospital mortality alter coronary artery bypass surgery: evidence for a higher mortality in younger women. *Circulation* 105: 1176–1181, 2002.

[175] Deshotels, A; Planchock, N; Dech, Z; *et al.* Gender differences in perception of quality of life in cardiac rehabilitation patients. *J Cardiopulm Rehabil.* 15(2): 143-148, 1995.

[176] Wamala, SP; Lynch, J, and Kaplan, GA. Women's exposure to early and later life socio-economic disadvantage and coronary heart disease risk: the Stockholm Female Coronary Risk Study. *Int J Epidemiol.* 30: 275–284, 2001.

[177] Prescott, E; Holst, C; Gronbaek, M; *et al.*Vital exhaustion as a risk factor for ischemic heart disease and all-cause mortality in a community sample. A prospective study of 4,084 men and 5,479 women in the Copenhagen City heart study. *Int J Epidemiol.* 32: 990-997, 2003.

[178] Brezinka, V, and Kittel, F. Psychosocial factors of coronary heart disease in women: a review. *Soc Sci Med.* 42:1351–1365, 1996.

[179] Fleury, J; Sedikides, C, and Lunsford, V. Women's experience following a cardiac event: the role of the self in healing. *J Cardiovasc Nurs.* 15(3): 71-82, 2001.

[180] Hagbert, V; Sjöberg, T, and Ivarsson, B. Older women with a serious cardiac event experience support with a Vifladt & Hopen inspired patient group education programme. *Eur J of Cardiovasc Nurs.* 7: 140-146, 2008.

[181] Westin, L; Carlsson, R; Erhardt, L ; *et al.* Differences in quality of life in men and women with ischemic heart disease. A prospective controlled study. *Scand Cardiovasc J.* 33(3): 160-165, 1999.

[182] Todaro, JF; Shen, BJ, and Niaura, R. Do men and women achieve similar benefits from cardiac rehabilitation? *J Cardiopulm Rehabil.* 24(1): 45-51, 2004.

[183] Leon, AS; Franklin, BA; Costa, F; *et al.* Cardiac rehabilitation and secondary prevention of coronary heart disease; an American Heart Association scientific statement from the Council on Clinical Cardiology (subcommittee on exercise, cardiac rehabilitation and prevention) and the Council on Nutrition, Physical Activity and Metabolism (subcommittee on physical activity), in collaboration with the American Association of Cardiovascular and Pulmonary Rehabilitation. *Circulation* 111: 369-376, 2005.

[184] Claesson, M; Birgander, LS; Lindahl, B; et al. Women's hearts—stress management for women with ischemic heart disease. *J Cardiopulm Rehabil.* 25: 93-102, 2005.

[185] Barbour, KA; Edenfield, TM., and Blumenthal, JA, Exercise as a treatment for depression and other psychiatric disorders *J Cardiopulm Rehabil Prevent* 27: 359– 367, 2007.

[186] Dinnes, J. Cardiac rehabilitation. *Nurs Times* 94(38): 50-51, 1998.

[187] Higginson, R. Women are neglected when it comes to cardiac rehabilitation. *Br J Nurs* 12(12): 713, 2003.

[188] Mitchell, R; Muggli, M, and Sato A. Cardiac rehabilitation: participating in an exercise programs in a quest to survive. *Rehabil Nurs.* 24(6): 236-270, 1999.

[189] Parks, D; Allison, M; Doughty, R; et al. An audit of phase II cardiac rehabilitation at Auckland hospital. *NZMJ* 113: 158-161, 2000.

[190] Evans, L; Probert, H, and Shuldham, C. Cardiac rehabilitation past to present *J Res Nurs.* 14: 223- 240, 2009.

[191] Lavie, C, and Milani, R. Effects of cardiac rehabilitation and exercise training on exercise capacity, coronary risk factors, behavioral characteristics, and quality of life in women. *Am J Cardiol.* 75: 340-343, (Feb. 1995).

[192] Fridlund, B. Self-related health in women after their first myocardial infarction: A 12 month comparison between participation and nonparticipation in a cardiac rehabilitation program. *Hlth Care Women Int.* 21: 727-738, 2000.

[193] Goldberg, RJ; McCormick, D; Gurwitz, JH; et al. Age-related trends in short- and long-term survival after acute myocardial infarction: a 20 year population-based perspective. *Am J Cardiol.* 82:1311-1317, 1998.

[194] Ades, P; Waldermann, M; Polk, D; et al. Referral patterns and exercise response in the rehabilitation of female coronary patients aged ≥ 62 years. *Am J of Cardiology* 69: 1422-1425, 1992.

[195] Witt, BJ ; Jacobsen, SJ ; Weston, SA ; et al. Cardiac rehabilitation after myocardial infarction in the community. *J Am Coll Cardiol.* 44: 988–996, 2004.

[196] Cortes, O, and Arthur, HM. Determinants of referral to cardiac rehabilitation programs in patients with coronary artery disease: a systematic review. *Am Heart J.* 151: 249–256, 2006.

[197] Suaya, JA; Shepard, DS; Normand, SL; et al. Use of cardiac rehabilitation by Medicare beneficiaries after myocardial infarction or coronary bypass surgery. *Circulation* 116(15):1653–1662, 2007.

[198] Stewart, DE ; Abbey, SE, Shnek, ZM ; *et al.* Gender differences in health information needs and decisional preferences in patients recovering from an acute ischemic coronary event. *Psychosom Med* 66: 42–48, 2004.

[199] Worcester, MUC; Murphy, BM; Mee, VK; *et al.* Cardiac rehabilitation programmes: predictors of non-attendance and drop-out. *Eur J Cardiovasc Prev Rehabil.* 11: 328–335, 2004.

[200] Bjarnason-Wehrens, B; Grande, G; Loewel, H; *et al.* Gender-specific issues in cardiac rehabilitation: do women with ischemic heart disease need specially tailored programmes? *Eur J Cardiovasc Prev Rehabil.* 14: 163-171, 2007.

[201] New Zealand Guideliness Group (NZGG) and New Zealand Heart Foundation. Best practice evidence-based guideliness– cardiac rehabilitation 2002. Available at: *http://www.nzgg.org.nz/guideliness/0001/Summary_resource_kit.pdf.* Accessed: 25 August 2006.

[202] Stone, JA, and Arthur, HM. Canadian guidelines for cardiac rehabilitation and cardiovascular disease prevention, 2nd ed. 2004: Executive summary. *Can J Cardiol.* 21(suppl D):3D-19D, 2005.

[203] American Association of Cardiovascular and Pulmonary Rehabilitation. Guidelines for cardiac rehabilitation and secondary prevention programs. Champaign: Human Kinetics, 2005

[204] Wenger, NK; Froelicher, ES; Smith, LK; *et al.* Cardiac rehabilitation as secondary prevention. Agency for Health Care Policy and Research and National Heart, Lung, and Blood Institute. *Clin Pract Guidel Quick Ref Guide Clin.* 17: 1-23, 1995.

[205] Scottish Guidelines Intercollegiate Network (SIGN). Cardiac rehabilitation. A national clinical guideline. SIGN publication no. 57. Edinburgh: SIGN, 2002.

[206] Balady, GJ; Williams, MA; Ades, PA ; *et al.* Core components of cardiac rehabilitation/secondary prevention programs: 2007 update. A scientific statement from the American Heart Association Exercise, Cardiac Rehabilitation, and Prevention Committee, the Council on Clinical Cardiology; the Councils on Cardiovascular Nursing, Epidemiology and Prevention, and Nutrition, Physical Activity, and Metabolism; and the American Association of Cardiovascular and Pulmonary Rehabilitation. *Circulation* 115: 2675-2682, 2007.

[207] Hamalainen, H ; Luurila, OJ ; Kallio, V ; *et al.* Reduction in sudden deaths and coronary mortality in myocardial infarction patients after

rehabilitation. 15 year follow-up study. *Eur Heart J.* 16: 1839- 1844, 1995.

[208] Burrowes, JD. Preventing heart disease in women. *Nutr Today* 42(6): 242-247, 2007.

[209] U.S. Department of Health and Human Services: Physical activity and health: a report of Surgeon General. In Atlanta, GA: Centers of Disease Control and Prevention, National Center for Chronic Disease Prevention and Health Promotion, 1996.

[210] Centers for Disease Control and Prevention Web site, Physical activity and health. U.S. Department of Health and Human Services. Available at: *www.cdc.gov/nccdphp/sgr/women* (Accessed April 24, 2008)

[211] U.S. Department of Health and Human Services. Healthy People 2010: Understanding and improving health. Washington, DC: U.S. Government Printing Office, 2000.

[212] Moore, SM; Ruland, CM; Pashkow, FJ; *et al.* Women's patterns of exercise following cardiac rehabilitation. *Nurs Res.* 47(6): 318- 324, 1998.

[213] Moore, SM; Dolansky, MA; Ruland, CM; *et al.* Predictors of women's exercise maintenance after cardiac rehabilitation. *J Cardiopulm Rehabil.* 23: 40-49, 2003.

[214] Koffman, DM; Bazzare, T; Mosca, L; *et al.* An evaluation of choose to move 1999; an American Heart Association physical activity program for women. *Arch Intern Med.* 161: 2193-2199, 2001.

[215] Pazoki, R; Nabipour, I; Seyednezami, N; *et al.* Effects of a community-based heart program on increasing healthy women's physical activity: a randomized controlled trial guided by Community-based Participatory Research (CBPR) BMC *Public Hlth.* 7: 216, 2007. doi: 10.1186/1471-2458-7-216.

[216] Beckie, TM. A behavior change intervention for women in cardiac rehabilitation. *J Cardiovasc Nurs.* 21(2): 146-153, 2006.

[217] Durstine, JL, and Haskell, WL. Effects of exercise training on plasma lipid and lipoproteins. *Exerc Sport Sci Rev.* 22: 477-521, 1994.

[218] Williams, PT. High-density lipoprotein cholesterol and other risk factors for coronary heart disease in female runners. *N Eng J Med.* 334: 1298-1303, 1996.

[219] Stewart, KJ; Turner, KL; Bacher, AC; *et al.* Are fitness, activity, and fatness associated with health-related quality of life and mood in older persons? *J Cardiopulm Rehabil.* 23(2):115-121, 2003.

[220] Taylor, RS; Brown, A; Ebrahim, S; *et al.* Exercise-based rehabilitation for patients with coronary heart disease: systematic review and meta-analysis of randomized controlled trials. *Am J Med.* 116: 682-692, 2004.

[221] Kushi, LH; Fee, RM; Folsom, AR; *et al.* Physical activity and mortality in postmenopausal women. *JAMA* 277: 1287-1292, 1997.

[222] Rockhill, B ; Willett, WC ; Manson, JE ; *et al.* Physical activity and mortality: a prospective study among women. *Am J Public Health* 91: 578-583, 2001.

[223] Wood, PD; Stefanick, ML; Williams, PT; *et al.* The effects of on plasma lipoproteins of a prudent weight-reducing diet, with or without exercise, in overweight men and women. *N Eng J Med.* 325: 461-466, 1991.

[224] Troisi, RJ; Heinhold, JW; Vokonas, PS ; *et al.* Cigarette smoking, dietary intake, and physical activity: effects on body fat distribution- The Normative Aging Study. *Am J Clin Nutr.* 11: 1250-1257, 1991.

[225] Wing, RR; Matthews, KA; Kuller, LH; *et al.* Waist to hip ratio in middle aged women. Associations with behavioral and psychosocial factors and what changes in cardiovascular risk factors. *Arterioscler Thromb* 11: 1250-1257, 1991.

[226] Kisioglu, AN; Aslan, B; Ozturk, M; *et al.* Improving control of high blood pressure among middle-aged Turkish women of low socioeconomic status through public health training. *CMJ* 45(4): 477-482, 2004

[227] Paffenbarger, RS; Hyde, RT; Wing, A; *et al.* Physical activity, all-cause mortality, and longevity of college of alumni. *N Eng J Med.* 314: 605-613, 1986.

[228] Manson, JE; Stampfer, MJ; Colditz, GA; *et al.* A prospective study of exercise and incidence of myocardial infarction in women. *Circulation* 88: 1-220, 1993.

[229] Leon, A; Connett, J; Jacobs, DR; *et al.* Leisure time physical activity levels and risk of coronary heart disease and death. The multiple risk factor intervention trial. *JAMA* 258: 2388-2395, 1987.

[230] Halm, M, and Denker, J. Primary prevention programs to reduce heart disease risk in women. *Clin Nurse Specialist* 17(2): 101-109, 2003.

[231] Asikainen, TM; Kukkonen-Harjula, K, and Milunpalo, S. Exercise for health for early postmenopausal women: a systematic review of randomized controlled trials. *Sports Med.* 34: 753–778, 2004.

[232] Oldridge, NB; Guyatt, GH; Fischer, ME; *et al.* Cardiac rehabilitation after myocardial infarction: combined experience of randomized clinical trials. *JAMA* 260: 945–950, 1988.

[233] O'Connor, GT; Buring, JE; Yusuf, S; *et al.* An overview of randomized trials of rehabilitation with exercise after myocardial infarction. *Circulation* 80: 234–244, 1989.

[234] Williams, MA; Ades, PA; Hamm, LF; *et al.* Clinical evidence for a health benefit from cardiac rehabilitation: an update. *Am Heart J.* 152: 835-841, 2006.

[235] Naughton, J; Dorn, J, and Imamura, D. Outcomes measurement in cardiac rehabilitation: the national exercise and heart disease project. *J Rehabild Outcomes Measur* 4(4): 64-75, 2000.

[236] Conn, VS; Taylor, SG, and Casey, B. Cardiac rehabilitation program participation and outcomes after myocardial infarction. *Rehabil Nurs* 17(2)58-63, 1992.

[237] Claesson, M; Burell, G; Birgander, LS; *et al.* Psychosocial distress and impaired quality of life – targets neglected in the secondary prevention in women with ischemic heart disease. *Eur J Cardiovasc Prev Rehabil.* 10: 258-266, 2003.

[238] Lau, J; Antman, EM; Jimenez-Silva, □ ; *et al.* Cumulative meta-analysis of therapeutic trials for myocardial infarction. *N Eng J Med.* 327.248-254, 2002.

[239] Jolliffe, JA; Rees, K; Taylor, RS; *et al.* Exercise based rehabilitation for coronary heart disease. Cochrane Database System Revision 2001; 1: CD001800.

[240] Clark, AM; Hartling, L; Vandermeer, B; *et al.* Meta-analysis: secondary prevention programs for patients with coronary artery disease. *Ann Intern Med.* 143: 659-672, 2005.

[241] Oldridge, NB; LaSalle, D, and Jones, NL. Exercise rehabilitation of female patients with coronaryheart disease. *Am Heart J.* 100: 755-757, 1980.

[242] Bittner, V, and Sanderson, BK. Women in cardiac rehabilitation. *JAMWA* 58: 227-235, 2003.

[243] Kennedy, MD; Haykowsky, M; Daub, B; *et al.* Effects of a comprehensive cardiac rehabilitation program on quality of life and exercise tolerance in vomen: a retrospective analysis. *Curr Control Trials Cardiovasc Med.* 4: 1, 2003.

[244] O'Farrel, P; Murray, J; Huston, P; *et al.* Sex differences in cardiac rehabilitation. *Can J Cardiol.* 16: 319-325, 2000.

[245] Verrill, D; Barton, C; Beasley, W; *et al.* Quality of life measures and gender comparisons in North Carolina Cardiac Rehabilitation Programs. *J Cardiopulm Rehabil.* 21: 37-46, 2001.

[246] Balady, GJ; Jette, D; Scheer, J ; *et al.* Changes in exercise capacity following cardiac rehabilitation in patients stratified according to age and gender. Results of Massachusetts Association of Cardiovascular and Pıulmonary Rehabilitation Multicenter Database. *J Cardiopulm Rehabil.* 16; 38-46, 1996.

[247] Savage, PD; Brochu, M, and Ades, PA. Gender alters the high-density lipoprotein cholesterol response to cardiac rehabilitation *J Cardiopulm Rehabil.* 24: 248-256, 2004.

[248] Gupta, R; Sanderson, BK, and Bittner, V. Outcomes at one-year follow-up of women and men with coronary artery disease discharged from cardiac rehabilitation. What benefits are maintained? *J Cardiopul Rehabil Prev.* 27: 11-18, 2007.

[249] Allen, JK. Coronary risk factors in women one year after coronary artery bypass grafting. *J Womens Health Gend Based Med.* 8: 617-622, 1999.

[250] Robiner, WN. Enhancing adherence in clinical research. *Contemp Clin Trials* 26:59-77, 2005.

[251] Roter, DL; Hall, JA; Merisca, R; *et al.* Effectiveness of interventions to improve patient compliance: a meta-analysis. *Medical Care* 36: 1138-1161, 1998.

[252] McDonald, HP; Garg, AX, and Haynes, RB. Interventions to enhance patient adherence to medication prescriptions: scientific review. *JAMA* 288: 2868-2879, 2002.

[253] Cooper, A; Lioyd, G; Weinman, J; *et al.* Why patients do not attend cardiac rehabilitation: role of intentions and beliefs. *Heart* 82: 234-246, 1999.

[254] Petrie, KJ; Weinman, J; Sharpe, N; *et al.* Role of patients' view of their illness in predicting return to work and functioning after myocardial infarction: longitudinal study. *BMJ* 312: 1191-1194, 1996.

[255] Low, KG; Thoresen, CE; Pattillo, JR; *et al.* Causal attributions and coronary heart disease in women. *Psychol Rep.* 73. 627-636, 1993.

[256] Astin, F, and Jones, K. Heart disease attributions of patients prior to elective percutaneous transluminal coronary angioplasty. *J Cardiovasc Nurs.* 19: 41-47, 2004.

[257] Furze, G, and Lewin, B. Causal attributions for angina: results of an interview study. *Coron Health Care* 4: 130-134, 2000.

[258] Halm, M; Penque, S; Doll, N; *et al.* Women and cardiac rehabilitation: Referral and compliance patterns. *J Cardiovasc Nurs.* 13(3): 83-92, 1999.

[259] Gallagher, R; McKinley, S, and Dracup, K. Predictors of women's attendance at cardiac rehabilitation programs. *Prog Cardiovasc Nurs.* 18: 121-126, 2003.

[260] Schuster, PM; Wright, C, and Tomich, P. Gender differences in the outcomes of participants in home programs compared to those in structured cardiac rehabilitation programs. *Rehabil Nurs.* 20: 93-101, 1995.

[261] Jackson, L; Leclerc, J; Erskine, Y ; *et al.* Getting the most of out cardiac rehabilitation; a review of referral and adherence predictors. *Heart* 91: 10-14, 2005.

[262] Scott, IA; Eyeson-Annan, ML; Huxley, SL; *et al.* Optimizing care of acute myocardial infarction; results of a regional quality improvement project. *J Qual Clin Pract.* 20: 12-19, 2000.

[263] Parsk, D; Allison, M; Doughty, R ; *et al.* An audit of phase II cardiac rehabilitation at Auckland hospital. *NZ Med J.* 113: 158-161, 2000.

[264] Evans, JA; Turner, SC, and Bethell, HJN. Cardiac rehabilitation: are the NSF milestones achievable. *Heart* 87 (Suppl) II: 41, 2002.

[265] Scott, LB, and Allen, JK. Providers' perceptions of factors affecting women's referral to outpatient cardiac rehabilitation programs: an exploratory study. *J Cardiopulm Rehabil.* 24: 387–391, 2004.

[266] Jeger, RV; Jorg, L; Rickenbacher, P; *et al.* Benefit of outpatient cardiac rehabilitation in under-represented patient subgroups. *J Rehabil Med.* 39: 246–251, 2007.

[267] Ades, PA; Waldmann, ML; McCann, WJ; *et al.* Predictors of cardiac rehabilitation participation in older coronary patients. *Arch Intern Med.* 152:1033-1035, 1992.

[268] Oldridge, NB; Ragowski, B, and Gottlieb, M. Use of outpatient cardiac rehabilitation services. Factors associated with attendance. *J Cardiopulm Rehabil.* 12: 25-31, 1992.

[269] Anderson, GL; Limacher, M; Assaf, AR ; *et al.* Effects of conjugated equine estrogen in postmenopausal women with hysterectomy: the Women's Health Initative randomized controlled trial. *JAMA* 291: 1701-1712, 2004.

[270] Rossow, JE; Prentice, RL; Manson, JE; *et al.* Postmenopausal hormone therapy and risk of cardiovascular disease by age and years since menopause. *JAMA* 297: 1465-1477, 2007.

[271] Jacobs, AK. Coronary revascularization in women in 2003. Sex revisited. *Circulation* 107: 375, 2003.

[272] Thomas, RJ; Miller, NH; Lamendola, C; *et al.* National survey on gender differences in cardiac rehabilitation programs: patient characteristics and enrollment patterns. *J Cardiopul Rehabil.* 16 (6): 25-31, 1996.

[273] Daly, J; Sindone, AP; Thompson, DR; *et al.* Barriers to participation in and adherence to cardiac rehabilitation programs: a critical literature review. *Prog Cardiovasc Nurs.* 17: 8-17, 2002.

[274] Caulin-Glaser, T; Maciejewski, PK; Snow, R; *et al.* Depressive symptoms and sex affect completion rates and clinical outcomes in cardiac rehabilitation. *Prev Cardiol.* 10: 15-21, 2007.

[275] Yohannes, AM; Yalfani, A; Doherty, P; *et al.* Predictors of drop-out from an outpatient cardiac rehabilitation program. *Clin Rehabil.* 21: 222-229, 2007.

[276] Harrison, WN, and Wardle, SA. Factors affecting the uptake of cardiac rehabilitation services in a rural locality. *Public Hlth.* 119: 1016-1022, 2005.

[277] Weiss, BD. Diagnostic evaluation of urinary incontinence in geriatric patients. *Am Family Physician* 57: 2675-2684; 2688-2690, 1998.

[278] Nihira, MA, and Henderson, N. Epidemiology of urinary incontinence in women. *Curr Womens Hlth Rep.* 3: 340-347, 2003.

[279] Marchionni, N; Fattirolli, F; Fumagalli, S ; *et al.* Improved exercise tolerance and quality of life with cardiac rehabilitation of older patients after myocardial infarction results of a randomized, controlled trial. *Circulation* 107: 2201-2206, 2003.

[280] Hasmen, P; Ceci, R, and Backman, L. Exercise for older women: A training method and its influences on physical and cognitive performance. *Eur J Appl Physiol Occup Physiol.* 64: 460-466, 1992.

[281] Barefoot, JC; Burmmett, BH; Helms, MJ; *et al.* Depressive symptoms and survival of patients with coronary artery disease. *Psychosom Med.* 62: 790-795, 2000.

[282] Glazer, KM; Emery, CF; Frid, DJ; *et al.* Psychological predictors of adherence and outcomes among patients in cardiac rehabilitation. *J Cardiopulm Rehabil.* 22: 40-46, 2002.

[283] Ziegelstein, R; Fauerbach, J; Stevens, S; *et al.* Patients with depression are less likely to follow recommendations to reduce cardiac risk during recovery from a myocardial infarction. *Arch Intern Med.* 160: 1818-1823, 2000.

[284] Lichtman, JH; Bigger, JT; Blumenthal, JA; *et al.* Depression and coronary heart disease: recommendations for screening, referral, and

treatment: a science advisory from the American Heart Association Prevention Committee of the Council on Cardiovascular Nursing, Council on Clinical Cardiology, Council on Epidemiology and Prevention, and Interdisciplinary Council on Quality of Care and Outcomes Research: Endorsed by the American Psychiatric Association. *Circulation* 118; 1768-1775, 2008.

[285] Le Bourdais, C; Hamel, PJ, and Bernard, P. Le travail et l'ouvrage. Charge at partage des taches domestiques chez les couples quebecois. *Sociol Soc* 19. 37-55, 1987.

[286] Wright, EO; Shire, K; Hwang, S-L; *et al.* The noneffects of class on the gender division of labor in the home: a comparative study of Sweden and the United States. *Gender Soc* 6(2): 252-282, 1992.

[287] Biernat, M, and Wortman, CB. Sharing of home responsibilities between professionally employed women and their husbands. *J Pers Soc Psychol.* 60:844-860, 1991.

[288] Lane, D; Carroll, D; Ring, C; *et al.* Predictors of attendance at cardiac rehabilitation after myocardial infarction. *J Psychosomatic Res.* 51: 497-501, 2001

[289] Lee, S; Colditz, GA; Berkman, LF; *et al.* Caregiving and risk of coronary heart disease in us women. *Am J Prev Med.* 24(2): 113-119, 2003.

[290] Walters, W. The social context of women's health. *BMC Women's Hlth.* 4:S2, 2004.

[291] Cohen, PN, and Bianchi, SM. Marriage, children, and women's employment: what do we know? *Mthly Labor Rev.* pp. 22–31, (December 1999).

[292] Hall, EM. Gender, work control, and stress: a theoretical discussion and an empirical test. *Int J Hlth Serv* 19(4): 725-745, 1989.

[293] Laflamme, N; Brisson, C; Moisan, J ; *et al.* Job strain and ambulatory blood pressure among female white-collar workers. *Scand J Work Environ Hlth.* 24: 334-343, 1998.

[294] Verlander, G. Female physicians: balancing career and family. *Acad Psychiatry* 28: 331-336, 2004.

[295] Lieberman, L; Meana, M, and Stewart, D. Cardiac rehabilitation: gender differences in factors influencing participation. *J Womens Hlth.* 7: 717-723, 1998.

[296] Allen, JK; Scott, LB; Stewart, KJ; *et al.* Disparities in women's referral to and enrollment in outpatient cardiac rehabilitation. *J Gen Intern Med* 19: 747-753, 2004.

[297] Evenson, KR; Rosamond, WD, and Luepker, RV. Predictors of outpatient cardiac rehabilitation utilization: the Minnesota Heart Surgery Registry. *J Cardiopulm Rehabil.* 18: 192-198, 1998.

[298] Johnson, SM; Karvonen, CA; Phelps, CL; *et al.* Assessment of analysis by gender in the Cochrane reviews as related to treatment of cardiovascular disease. *J Womens Hlth (Larchmt)* 12: 449-457, 2003.

[299] Husak, L; Krumholz, HM; Lin, ZQ; *et al.* Social support as a predictor of participation in cardiac rehabilitation after coronary bypass graft surgery *J Cardiopulm Rehabil.* 24: 19-26, 2004.

[300] Caulin-Glaser, T; Blum, M; Schmeizl, R; *et al.* Gender differences in referral to cardiac rehabilitation programs after revascularization. *J Cardiopulm Rehabil.* 21: 24-30, 2001.

[301] Apple, LJ; Moore, TJ; Obarzanek, E ; *et al.* A clinical trial of the effects of dietary patterns on blood pressure, DASH Collaborative Research Group, *N Engl J Med.* 336: 1117-1124, 1997.

[302] Parkosewich, JA. Cardiac rehabilitation barriers and opportunities among women with cardiovascular disease. *Cardiol Rev.* 16: 36-52, 2008.

[303] Evenson, KR, and Fleury, J. Barriers to outpatient cardiac rehabilitation participation and adherence. *J Cardiopulm Rehabil.* 20: 241-246, 2000.

[304] Farley, RL; Wade, TD, and Birchmore, L. Factors influencing attendance at cardiac rehabilitation among coronary heart disease patients. *Eur J Cardiovasc Nurs.* 2: 205-212, 2003.

[305] Grace, SL; Evindar, A; Brooks, D; *et al.* Increasing patient initiation of cardiac rehabilitation referral in female percutaneus coronary intervention patients. *Can J Cardiovasc Nurs.* 15: 23-27, 2005.

[306] Heidi, HG, and Schmelzer, M. Influences on women's participation in cardiac rehabilitation. *Rehabil Nurs.* 29: 116-121, 2004.

[307] Grace, SL; Scholey, P; Suskin, N; *et al.* A prospective comparison of cardiac rehabilitation enrollment following automatic vs usual referral. *J Rehabil Med.* 39: 239-245, 2007.

[308] Harkness, K; Smith, KM; Taraba, L; *et al.* Effect of a postoperative telephone intervention on attendance at intake for cardiac rehabilitation after coronary artery bypass graft surgery. *Heart Lung* 34: 179-186, 2005.

[309] Clark, AM; Barbour, RS; White, M; *et al.* Promoting participation in cardiac rehabilitation: patient choices and experiences. *J Adv Nurs.* 47: 5-14, 2004.

[310] Moore, SM. Women's views of cardiac rehabilitation programs. *J Cardiopulm Rehabil.* 16: 123-129, 1996.

[311] Cochrane, BL. Acute myocardial infarction in women. *Crit Care Clin N Am* 4: 279, 1992.

[312] Brown, V; Bryson, L; Byles, J; *et al.* Women's health Australia: Recruitment for a national longitudinal cohort study. *Women Hlth.* 28(1): 23-40, 1998.

[313] Marzolini, S; Brooks, D, and Oh, PI. Sex differences in completion of a 12-month cardiac rehabilitation programme: an analysis of 5,922 women and men. *Eur J Cardiovasc Prev Rehabil.* 15: 698–703, 2008.

[314] Filip, J; McGillen, C, and Mosca, L. Patient preferences for cardiac rehabilitation and desired program elements. *J Cardiopulm Rehabil.* 19: 339-343, 1999.

[315] Grace, SL; McDonald, J; Fishman, D ; *et al.* Patient preferences for home based versus hospital-based cardiac rehabilitation. *J Cardiopulm Rehabil.* 25: 24-29, 2005.

[316] Wingham, J; Dalal, HM; Sweeney, KG; *et al.* Listening to patients: choice in cardiac rehabilitation. *Eur J Cardiovasc Nurs.* 5: 289-294, 2006.

INDEX